StressMap®

PERSONAL DIARY EDITION

*The Ultimate
Stress Management,
Self-Assessment
and Coping Guide
Developed by Essi Systems*

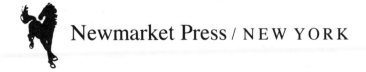

Newmarket Press / NEW YORK

StressMap is dedicated to the effort
for world peace.

This book published simultaneously in the
United States of America and in Canada.

10 9 8 7

Revisions for this expanded edition by Esther M. Orioli,
President of Essi Systems. The original *StressMap®* was co-authored by Esther
M. Orioli, M.S., Dennis T. Jaffe, Ph.D., and Cynthia D. Scott, Ph.D., M.P.H.

LIBRARY OF CONGRESS CATALOGING-IN-PUBLICATION DATA
StressMap: the ultimate stress management, self-assessment, and coping
guide/developed by Essi Systems.--Expanded personal diary ed.
p. cm.
Rev. ed. of: StressMap/
Esther M. Orioli, Dennis T. Jaffe, Cynthia D. Scott
Includes biographical references.
ISBN 1-55704-081-8
1. StressMap.   I. Orioli, Esther M. StressMap.
II. Essi Systems.
BF575.S75075   1991
155.9'042'0287--dc20   90-48965
                                                          CIP

QUANTITY PURCHASES
Companies, professional groups, clubs, and other organizations may qualify
for special terms when ordering quantities of this title.
For information, contact the Special Sales Department,
Newmarket Press, 18 East 48th Street,
New York, New York 10017, (212) 832-3575.

Book design by Helen Barrow
Manufactured in the United States of America

CONTENTS

Foreword

Mastering *Stress*—the nonstop pressures and demands of your work, family, and personal life—is one of the greatest challenges each of us must face, today and in the years ahead. But contrary to popular myth, stress itself is neither good nor bad; it's simply an energy force. Day in and day out, it can enhance—or break down—your health and performance. It all depends on how well you understand, and manage, its power and influence in your life.

Many of us are paying a serious price for mismanaged stress. It already costs American businesses an estimated $200 billion a year (which is more than the profits of all the *Fortune 500* companies combined). Nearly one-fifth of all occupational health claims are now for job stress—an increase of several hundred percent in only a few years. In addition, medical researchers estimate that stress is linked to 65 to 90 percent of all illnesses and diseases.

Scientists report that mismanaged stress affects the immune system, heart function, hormone levels, the nervous system, memory and thinking, physical coordination, and metabolic rate; it raises blood cholesterol, blood pressure, and uric acid levels; and it may increase the risk of certain diseases, including heart disease, cancer, immunodeficiency diseases, and even the common cold.

Every year, more than 500,000 Americans die from heart attacks—300,000 before reaching a hospital. A surprising number of these deaths (for both men and women) are due to what some cardiologists call *silent heart disease*—where the victims have none of the usual cardiac danger symptoms, such as high blood pressure, obesity, or elevated blood cholesterol. These people are often high achieving, physically fit, and healthy on the outside but have a time bomb tied to their hearts—*hidden stress* may be breaking down the heart muscle and creating a high risk of heart attack.

As the pace and complexity of life continue to increase, researchers worldwide are concluding that it's never been more critical to effectively manage the pressures you face at work and at home. One of the keys is finding—and taking better control of—your own stress hot spots: those specific demands and situations that trigger anxiety, anger, frustration, impatience, or physical signs such as shortness of breath, tightness in the chest or throat, yelling, clenched fists, mental distraction, or feelings of fatigue.

StressMap: Personal Diary Edition is one of the quickest and most accurate ways to measure your personal stress load. And then, once you identify any problem areas, this book offers some simple, straightforward advice for you to begin reducing distress and creating healthier responses to the difficult and challenging situations in your life.

StressMap is a sound and practical self-assessment guide that's more vital today than ever before.

Robert K. Cooper, Ph.D.,
author of *Health & Fitness Excellence*
and *The Performance Edge*

Introduction

We think you'll find that *StressMap* is not just another book about stress. It is a powerful tool that can help you change the way you think about stress and the role it plays in your life. It is a personal journey, guiding you to explore and understand how stress can harm or enhance your health. It evolved out of our commitment to the belief that the more you know about your body and how stress affects you, the more likely you will be to make lasting changes in your health.

You have in your hands the "personal diary" edition of Essi Systems' *StressMap*. Until 1987, *StressMap* was presented solely in a three-part program kit sold mainly through health-assistance groups in corporations, hospitals, and other institutions. Developed over a five-year research and testing period, *StressMap* proved so successful that we were encouraged to make it available for individual purchase at bookstores and other consumer outlets. Therefore, we began publishing this integrated, booklike version, which is similar in all respects to the original *StressMap,* except that the Interpretation section has been greatly expanded. This current edition has been further enlarged to include timely discussions on how changes in the world around us and in our own personal value systems can influence the stress levels in our lives.

StressMap is organized into three sections. The first, the *StressMap* Self-Scoring Questionnaire, can be completed in less than an hour. It will identify your stress factors on 21 scales related to your Environment, your Coping Responses, your Inner World, and your Signals of Distress. The second section, the *StressMap* Scoring Grid, will enable you to chart your scores on a continuum of four performance zones—Burnout, Strain, Balance, and Optimal. The third section, the *StressMap* Interpretation, will help to demystify stress for you. It will explain what your scores on the Questionnaire mean and will help you identify, learn, and practice new and more effective ways of taking care of yourself.

As a whole, *StressMap* can provide you with a surprising self-portrait, a "snapshot" of the state of your stress level at a particular time. It can help you discover which of your current stress-management efforts are working for you and which ones may need bolstering. It can help you learn to uncover your stress "hot spots" and pinpoint where you need to make changes, focusing on elements within your control and targeting skills and behaviors that you can alter.

From Peak Performance to Optimal Performance

Over the years, my colleagues and I, as health educators, management consultants, and psychologists, had independently observed and studied thousands of employees and professionals in their workplace. We saw that too many people were giving up too much power. Many employees told us they worried about stress and that they felt unable to keep themselves healthy. One example from a study released in the summer of 1990 from the California Institute of Workers Compensation cites a 700 percent increase in the number of mental stress claims between 1979 and 1989, and reveals that 9 out of 10 claimants received compensation. Furthermore, one of the two "causes" that were assessed as the dominant culprits was job pressure.

In response to the perceived level of job related stress, companies scrambled to build gymnasiums and health clubs, hoping that the less fit would rush to them daily. (They didn't.) We saw an amazing increase in the number of wellness clinics, aerobics classes, relaxation sessions, and deep-breathing lessons. Hundreds of stress "experts" materialized to heal the afflicted. At every turn, we saw the fear of stress driving people to seek the newest, latest, or best way of achieving a long life and a healthy body.

The frenzy provided a temporary distraction from the issues that urgently needed to be addressed: there needed to be a new paradigm for thinking about stress, and this thinking was the genesis of *StressMap*. We decided we wanted to help people shift their focus—away from "peak performance" and striving for perfection, and toward the healthier goals of balance and optimal performance.

We used to think that peak performance was the only road to excellence. We now know that optimal performance rather than peak performance is what we seek. In its move from athletics to the workplace and personal life, the idea of peak performance has been misinterpreted as a sustainable state of being. But take a look at the meaning of the word "peak." Webster's defines it as "the top, a point, a rare occurrence, an exception to the usual." It is not a place you stay for long once you arrive, because every excursion up is followed by a journey down. Athletes who strive for peak performance do so in the context of a carefully planned training program. They have days of rest, days of light training, and days on which they aim for "peak performance." They know that, taken to the extreme, the push for peak performance can lead to the opposite of desired performance, often resulting in burnout.

This training philosophy, based on respect for the natural ebb and flow of one's personal rhythms, can be transferred to professional and personal life outside of sports. At Essi Systems we use the words "optimal performance" and "balance" to describe the concepts of personal harmony and productivity that lead to excellence.

Balance is a state of effective coping that emphasizes the importance of achieving and maintaining a healthy personal rhythm. This rhythm is determined by you and you alone. How healthy you keep your body, the way you act in stressful situations, and your attitudes, beliefs, and values all work together to form your personal style of coping. This definition of balance may require you to discard more traditional notions of excellence.

Optimal performance represents an integrated state of ease, comparable to a play state. When under pressure, the optimal performer mobilizes and responds in sync with her or his current physical, emotional, and intellectual abilities. She or he can tap reserves of energy and intuitive power to meet challenges and demands for effective management.

We used to think all stress is bad for you. We now know that stress is the everyday wear and tear on your body as you respond to the people, places, and things in your life. It can be either positive or negative, depending on how you perceive it and how you react to it. Take a look at some of the stressors you experience each day. Do you see them as threats? Or do you see them as challenges—opportunities for learning and growth? If you see them as challenges, chances are you experience them as manageable or negotiable.

On the other hand, if you think they are threats, you're probably experiencing them as oppressive and confining. Negative stress tends to create a feeling of frustration, helplessness, and alienation.

Stress sets in motion the genetically programmed red alert known as the "fight or flight response," which readied our ancestors to face danger by fighting or fleeing. Your heart rate and blood pressure rise, your mouth becomes dry, your palms sweaty. The dangers we face today, however, can't usually be dealt with by fighting or fleeing. And since our bodies don't know whether these dangers are real or imagined, they respond to both in the same way. Frequently, in cases of chronic stress, they're dangers we've created in our minds with negative attitudes and feelings of helplessness, both factors that can adversely affect your health. According to Joan Borysenko, Ph.D., author of *Minding the Body, Mending the Mind,* "Immunological studies . . . reveal that the inability to feel in control of stress [helplessness], rather than the stressful event itself, is the most damaging to immunity.''

The key is to learn to see yourself in each potentially distressful situation as having recourse to action that will result in your intellectual, spiritual, or emotional growth. Watch what your mind and feelings are telling you throughout the day.

We used to think physical fitness alone provides adequate protection from chronic illness. We now know that the body, mind, emotions, and spirit all play essential, interrelated roles in keeping us well.

Physical fitness is a very important, though not a solitary, contributor to your overall health. Exercise keeps your body functioning at its best: your bones, muscles, brain, nerves, and glands all need a physical workout for optimal health. Regular exercise also increases blood circulation, gives you greater lung capacity (which gives you access to more oxygen and thus more energy), strengthens the heart, lowers the heart rate, and reduces the risk of heart attack and stroke. Combined with a low-fat, high-fiber diet, exercise will *help* keep you in top form. It also improves self-esteem and self-image and in doing so contributes to your mental and emotional well-being.

In recent decades, scientific studies have supported what certain people have known for years: your physical, mental, emotional, and spiritual selves are inseparable, and mental, emotional, and spiritual health are just as important in protecting you from chronic illness as diet and exercise. Feeling connected to yourself and to others and having a sense of purpose in life are important factors for optimal health. In addition, a positive attitude, a feeling of hope, and the ability to create the life you want for yourself are key ingredients for maintaining overall health.

We used to think people who know how to completely control their lives are more powerful. We now know that people who try to control everything around them are, paradoxically, less in control than those who are able to "go with the flow." At the mercy of their conditioned attitudes and responses to stressors in life, they need to dominate all situations, including those they cannot possibly control. When faced with problems in traffic and lines in banks and stores, controllers become angry and mistrustful of the motives of others around them. These people are, for the most part, Type A personalities. Research by Redford Williams, M.D., an internist and behavioral medicine specialist at Duke University Medical Center, has shown that it is not the driving ambition, but rather the hostile, cynical emotions of Type A personalities (and the resultant constant outflow of stress hormones) that put them at risk for heart attack.

True control in life comes from learning to recognize situations that we *can* act on to change, if we wish to, and from recognizing those over which we have no control. Our sense of control comes from within—we are able to choose the reaction we will have to a situation, rather than fall victim to conditioned negative attitudes and feelings.

How Essi Systems' StressMap Evolved

Since 1983, I had been striving through Essi Systems to find ways to introduce these principles of balance, self assessment, and self management into Employee Assistance Programs. Then, in March 1984, Essi Systems saw the opportunity to expand the usefulness of a little-known stress-assessment tool, which had been developed in 1982 at the Center for Health Enhancement at the UCLA School of Medicine. Working through a grant from the Robert Simon Foundation, the Center had been asked to research links between stress-related problems and illness in human beings. A review of the literature identified more than 75 different factors from a wide variety of disciplines related to stress. They narrowed these factors down to 32, seeking a comprehensive yet balanced assessment device. The device was called the Personal Stress Inventory (PSI, 1983) and was used professionally as a diagnostic instrument with patients in therapy groups and in classroom settings.

During the next 18 months, Essi Systems explored how to transform this valuable PSI from a professional's diagnostic tool into a layperson's *self*-assessment device that met our own objectives—that is, to create tools and programs that encourage self knowledge, self management, and self responsibility in the areas of stress and personal performance.

The first question we needed to answer concerned the current state of the stress-management market and the need in the workplace for a stress-management tool. Did American corporations need another stress assessment? Working cooperatively with the Washington Business Group on Health, under an agreement from the Office of Disease Prevention and Health Promotion of the U.S. Department of Health and Human Services, we set out to research the state of stress in U.S. corporations. We wanted to find out how the modern-day employer defined stress, how stress was manifested in the workplace, and if there was any need whatsoever for another stress-management product. As a small company, we knew it was important to listen and to avoid any preconceived notions of what should or shouldn't be. When all the interviews were over, we had several interesting findings.

When asked if they do something about stress in their company, nearly all of the 50 human resource professionals we interviewed responded by stating yes. Most directors of health programs were eager to tell us about their health fairs, brown-bag lunch series, medical exams, and hypertension clinics. However, almost all of the professionals we talked to doubted that those efforts would bring about viable long-term results.

Furthermore, Essi research showed that *the highest per capita expenditures for stress programs had been spent on the upper and executive levels of organizations.* Retreats, weekend yachting trips, expensive workshops, and medical/physical workouts were frequently mentioned. Employees lower on the organizational ladder had either limited or no access to stress-management programs.

It was clear that the definitions of stress being used—and the efforts being made to address it in the workplace—fell short of achieving a comprehensive solution. We then asked a variety of health-related professionals, "If you could design the 'perfect' stress-management tool to meet the most pressing needs of your organization, what would it look like?"

We learned that human resource professionals wanted a tool that was self contained, self scoring, and comprehensive. Employee Assistance Program professionals wanted something that could help individuals change their behaviors and could be used as a guide to improving lifestyle. Supervisors said that time was a factor and that the perfect tool would require no time off from work and could be completed in less than an hour at home or in the office without a computer, counselor, or calculator. Training specialists favored a training or teaching guide that they could use in groups or simply distribute. Their concern was that such a guide should offer solutions to problems and immediate feedback, without having to wait for a printout. Of course, budget-conscious professionals everywhere said this magnificent creation should carry a one-time cost of no more than 10 dollars per person, be reusable, and be able to be administered in 45 minutes at a brown-bag lunch series.

In responding to these needs of the workplace, we developed four different prototypes of this stress-assessment tool. Our final product had a unique look, a special feel, and a distinct mission. It used nontechnical language, measured strengths as well as weaknesses, included a complete interpretation of scoring results, and showcased it all in a visually appealing format. We named it Essi Systems' *StressMap.*

Product testing and research into the norms, reliability, and validity of *StressMap* were conducted with nearly 400 employees throughout 1984 and 1985. The following companies and organizations participated in the testing and feedback phases. We gratefully acknowledge their importance and thank them for their role: Apple Computers, Inc.; AT&T Information Systems; Blue Cross of California; Dean Witter Reynolds; Physis Health Club; Sullivan Intermediate School; The Hospice of San Francisco; and The Harbor Bay Club. (For more information about the validity testing and respondent demographics for *StressMap,* see the Appendix.)

Included among the more than 1500 companies, institutions, and hospitals that have used *StressMap,* are the State of Maine, the Coca-Cola Company, Georgia Power & Light, and Tufts University. Essi Systems also offers a StressMap Presenters' Certification Package for in-house corporate programs and Company Profiler Composite Reports. To bring *StressMap* to an even larger audience, we are now presenting this expanded version of the Personal Diary Edition.

Acknowledgments

There are several people to thank for their roles and contributions in making this edition possible.

I wish to thank Jack McTaggart, whose emphatic belief in the value of *StressMap* led to its timely introduction to Newmarket Press.

I wish to acknowledge Esther Margolis, Publisher and President of Newmarket Press, for her pioneering spirit and adaptability in breaking from traditional publishing strictures to bring you this powerful, and somewhat unorthodox, learning tool.

I wish to thank Robert Wiele and Peter Jensen of the Center for High Performance in Toronto, Canada, for their model of mental fitness; Robert K. Cooper of Advanced Excellence Systems for his contributions to the world of corporate health and fitness; Madeleine Denko and Rogene Baxter for revisions and modifications to this manuscript; and Karen Trocki, Director of Research, Essi Systems, for her on-going creativity and research genius.

Special thanks to Robert N. Beck, Linda Fay, Florence Garcia, Paul Ash, Sylvia Orioli, Ellen Stevenson, Sue Yeres, Keith Stevenson, Robert Bixler, Veronica Darmon, and Nina and John Orioli for their love, support, and encouragement in the creation of *StressMap*.

My deepest love and gratitude to Pan Haskins for being there time and again.

Finally, I'd like to thank my editors Theresa Burns, Keith Hollaman, and Susan Rosalsky, plus all the employees and organizations who were willing to join us in the initial testing of *StressMap,* and the hundreds of companies and organizations throughout the United States and Canada who continue to report their satisfaction.

Esther M. Orioli, PRESIDENT
Essi Systems, Inc.

I

The StressMap Self-Scoring Questionnaire

You are about to embark on a very special journey, one that centers uniquely on you, your environment, and the ways you relate to the people, places, and events in your life. It is a journey that will raise questions that you may have thought were unrelated to stress. That is the whole point.

Stress has a bad reputation in our society. We perceive it as the enemy lurking in the bushes; ambush is inevitable. A brief review of any daily paper or magazine will offer a barrage of scary stories: stress is linked to cancer; political figures and corporate moguls take their lives because they are under too much pressure. Stress has attracted so much media attention and has become such a widespread concern that in some circles it is rapidly replacing sex as the most talked-about subject in America. Well, almost.

What exactly is stress, and where does it come from? Think of stress as a rubber band, one that contracts and expands depending on the amount of pressure or force exerted on it. When the band is pulled tight there is a greater demand on its elasticity. When it is not being pulled, there is no demand and it stays limp. If the band is constantly stretched without any release or easing of the pressure, it will begin to show signs of damage and will fray. In time it will snap.

Stress is the everyday wear and tear on your body as you respond to the people, places, and things in your life. If you take good care of your body, and make occasional allowances for the added strains that accompany unique or one-time stressors, you can keep that wear and tear in check. If, however, your body is like a neglected car whose owner demands peak performance and thinks the gas tank is the only part that requires attention, then stress will show itself in a gradual but inexorable deterioration. The result will be more frequent breakdowns and reduced performance. As minor calls for repair are ignored, the damage becomes more serious. Though the sources of stress may be emotional, mental, or spiritual, its impact can almost always be seen in a person's physical state.

Unlike a car, the human body has a remarkable ability to regenerate itself and repair even the most severe injuries. The resilient body is a fighter and a lover of life, and one of the most sophisticated healers on the face of the earth. When you begin to understand the power of this healing energy, you will come to realize the importance of your mental attitude in staying healthy.

In helping you to understand how you can live a less stressful life, our first task is to examine your current attitude toward stress. Is stress a monster you fear, or do you believe that stress is a necessary and desirable part of your life? Here's a simple way to check this for yourself. On a sheet of paper, write the word "stress" and then write down as many words as come to mind. Don't stop to think about them. Brainstorm without judging or evaluating each word. After you have listed about 10 or 12 words, go back and look at each of them. Ask yourself whether each of those words carries a positive or negative connotation. Put a plus sign next to those you consider positive and a minus sign next to those you consider negative. Do you have more of one than the other? This will identify your attitude toward stress.

Although many people perceive stress as negative and try to avoid it, we at Essi Systems believe that stress is actually essential and beneficial. It is the basic ingredient in optimal performance and can be our strongest ally for leading stimulating, healthy, satisfying lives. Yet, when unregulated, uncontrolled, or ignored, stress can be harmful. A major step toward successful stress management is to find and maintain a state of balance between too much and too little.

Preparing to Take the Questionnaire

As you begin your personal exploration, be sure to allow at least 35 minutes of undisturbed time, with as few distractions as possible. Select an environment or work space that allows you to concentrate on your *StressMap* Questionnaire. Remember that the responses you give are uniquely your own. There is no perfect score and as you rate yourself you are likely to find that, as in most journeys, your path will go up and down.

You will find that the Questionnaire is divided into 4 distinct parts, covering 21 scales in all.

Part One: Your Environment/Pressures and Satisfactions looks at the changes, pressures, and satisfactions that are part of your everyday work and personal worlds. Scales 1–3 deal with your work environment; scales 4–6, your personal environment. Altogether, this part examines the relationship between satisfactions and pressures in your life and the level of activity and change in these worlds.

Part Two: Coping Responses/Assets and Liabilities explores six basic skills that help you manage stressful situations. Scales 7–12 will accurately show you whether your current coping styles help or hinder your efforts to manage stress effectively.

Part Three: The Inner World/Thoughts and Feelings measures six different internal thinking and feeling patterns. The way you think and feel about things, your attitudes, and your values influence your choices in dealing with stress. Scales 13–18 will help you explore whether the judgments you make work for you or cause greater internal conflict.

Part Four: Signals of Distress, Scales 19–21, reveals the degree to which you are hampered by physical, behavioral, or emotional symptoms that reflect chronic difficulty in managing life and work stress.

Answering the Questionnaire

USE YOUR BEST GUESS

Begin with Scale 1, Work Changes. Complete each scale by circling the number (3, 2, 1, or 0) in the column that best describes your response to each statement. In all cases except Scales 1 and 4, Work Changes and Personal Changes respectively, the directions will ask you to think about the last month in answering the questions on that scale. Scales 1 and 4 ask you to think about the last year. If you are uncertain as to when something occurred, use your best guess. It is more important to measure how stress affects you than to be chronologically correct.

ANSWER ALL QUESTIONS

Some questions ask whether you agree or disagree with a statement; others ask how often you act or think in a certain way. Answer each question as best you can. Don't leave any question unanswered. Work quickly and stick to your initial response. Try to be as honest with yourself as possible. Only you will see your *StressMap* scores. If you have trouble answering a question, think of how a friend or co-worker might rate you on that item.

MAKE SUBSTITUTIONS

If you are a full-time student, you may wish to substitute the words "schoolwork" or "studies" for "work" and "job" in the Work Changes scale and make the appropriate substitutions in the rest of the Environment scales. You may think of your teachers as your supervisor and new courses of study as new job responsibilities.

If you are retired, or have never been employed outside the home, you may wish to substitute "my current life activities" or "my predominant work" for the Environment questions regarding Work Changes, Work Pressures, and Work Satisfactions. If these substitutions feel inappropriate, simply skip Scales 1–3 and begin with Scale 4, Personal Changes.

If you are currently unemployed or temporarily disabled, you may wish to think of your usual work situation when you answer Work Changes, Work Pressures, and Work Satisfactions. Work Pressures may be difficult to answer, depending on your situation. You may wish to skip Scales 2 and 3 and resume with Scale 4. Do not wait to become employed before completing your *StressMap*. You can use this opportunity to discover your stress performance on all the other scales. You will then be in the unusual position of having a snapshot before and after a new job or after a period of time off. Take advantage of this, and use *StressMap* to help you feel more balanced in seeking work. Feeling distressed has a way of coming through in a job interview.

Remember there are no right or wrong answers. There is no time limit. You can always go back to reconsider an answer. Every scale has face validity, which means you can tell what the scale is supposed to measure by the questions you are asked. *StressMap* is not a test, and there are no trick questions. Everyone who completes *StressMap* will have a unique graph or rhythm representing that individual only. You might want to better your own scores, however, each time you use *StressMap*.

Adding Up Your Scores

On each scale, add up the face value of each vertical column of numbers you have circled, placing the total at the bottom of each column. Then add these numbers horizontally to get your total score for that scale. Write that total in the large circle to the right of the column totals. (Please refer to the sample.)

Directly above the large circle is a ruler or thermometer that is divided into four levels, or zones. Your score from the large circle will fall into one of these zones. Locate the zone that corresponds to your score, and fill in the dot in that level.

Do this for each of the 21 scales. When you are ready, go to the *StressMap* Scoring Grid to complete your profile.

The *StressMap* Interpretation section will explain your results.

PART ONE
Your Environment/Pressures and Satisfactions

SCALE 1: Work Changes

Think about . . . the past **year**. *For each of the changes listed below, indicate how much or how little each has been a source of stress to you.*

	Great	Moderate	Little	None/Didn't Occur
New job or employer	3	2	1	0
New type of work	3	2	1	0
Change in work location or conditions	3	2	1	0
Change in responsibilities (promotion, demotion, or transfer)	3	2	1	0
Fired, laid off, quit, or retired	3	2	1	0
Passed over for promotion	3	2	1	0
Change in expectations, supervisors, or job role	3	2	1	0
New technologies or new management team/owner	3	2	1	0
Major new or special project or responsibility ...	3	2	1	0

0-2 ○
3-8 ○
9-13 ○
14+ ○

____ + ____ + ____ + ____ = ◯

Scale 1 Total

SCALE 2: Work Pressures

Think about . . . the past **month**. *For each of the pressures listed below, indicate how much each has been a source of stress to you.*

	Great	Moderate	Little	None
Workplace is bleak, uncomfortable, or depressing	3	2	1	0
Physically difficult or hazardous work conditions	3	2	1	0
Difficult or long commute	3	2	1	0
Too many job tasks and responsibilities	3	2	1	0
Boring routine tasks	3	2	1	0
Confused or unclear expectations	3	2	1	0
Conflicting or competing demands	3	2	1	0
No clear opportunities for promotion	3	2	1	0
Can't get the resources (information, help) I need for my work	3	2	1	0
Deadline pressures	3	2	1	0
Many organizational or job task changes	3	2	1	0
No input on decisions affecting my work	3	2	1	0
Responsibility for others	3	2	1	0
No recognition for work well done	3	2	1	0
Too many people telling me what to do	3	2	1	0
Office politics	3	2	1	0
Not sure where I stand with my supervisor	3	2	1	0
Pressured by demands from clients/customers . . .	3	2	1	0
Don't like my job	3	2	1	0
Job doesn't use my skills and abilities	3	2	1	0
No room for creativity or personal input	3	2	1	0
Ethical problems with my work	3	2	1	0
Have not gotten what I expected/wanted from my job	3	2	1	0
Loss of commitment or dedication to work	3	2	1	0
Inadequate salary	3	2	1	0
Conflict with co-workers or supervisor	3	2	1	0
Procedures are unfair or discriminatory	3	2	1	0
Too much or too little contact with people	3	2	1	0

```
____    ____    ____    ____

      +       +       +       =
____    ____    ____    ____
```

0-9 ○
10-19 ○
20-33 ○
34+ ○

○

Scale 2 Total

SCALE 3: Work Satisfactions

Think about . . . the past **month**. *For each of the satisfactions listed below, indicate how true each is for you.*

	Very	Somewhat	Little	Not At All
I enjoy my job	3	2	1	0
I like what my company or employer stands for	3	2	1	0
I have good relationships with people	3	2	1	0
I have a supervisor whom I like and trust	3	2	1	0
I have a good physical working environment	3	2	1	0
I receive adequate compensation for my work. . .	3	2	1	0
I am able to get the information I need to do my job	3	2	1	0
I feel liked and valued by the people at work	3	2	1	0
My work offers me the opportunity for advancement and growth	3	2	1	0
I receive feedback about the quality of my work	3	2	1	0
I use my abilities and talent on the job	3	2	1	0
The commute to my job is easy	3	2	1	0
The hours of work are convenient to my needs . .	3	2	1	0
I participate in decisions about things at work that affect me	3	2	1	0
I am respected by others in the community for my job	3	2	1	0

38 + ◯
32-37 ◯
24-31 ◯
0-23 ◯

____ + ____ + ____ + ____ = ◯

Scale 3 Total

NOTE: The term *family* is used generically to mean those people closest to you, your inner circle, and not necessarily a traditional family. The word *mate* is used generically to mean spouse, significant other, or life partner.

SCALE 4: Personal Changes

Think about . . . the past **year**. *For each of the changes listed below, indicate how much each has been a source of stress to you.*

	Great	Moderate	Little	None/ Didn't Occur
Change in residence	3	2	1	0
Death of a close family member or friend	3	2	1	0
Crisis with friend/family member (drug problem, job loss)	3	2	1	0
Separation or divorce of family member	3	2	1	0
A new close relationship	3	2	1	0
Your separation or divorce	3	2	1	0
Home improvement or repair	3	2	1	0
Illness or injury keeping you at home for a week or more	3	2	1	0
Change in family activities...................	3	2	1	0
New family member (birth, adoption)	3	2	1	0
Serious illness in family	3	2	1	0
Financial loss or diminished income	3	2	1	0
Major personal achievement	3	2	1	0
A major purchase or new debt	3	2	1	0
A "falling out" in a family or friendship	3	2	1	0
Involvement in legal system	3	2	1	0
Property loss, theft, damage, or accident	3	2	1	0
Crime victim.................................	3	2	1	0

____ + ____ + ____ + ____ =

0-4 ○
5-10 ○
11-18 ○
19+ ○

○
Scale 4 Total

SCALE 5: Personal Pressures

Think about . . . the past **month**. *For each of the pressures listed below, indicate how much each has been a source of stress to you.*

	Great	Moderate	Little	None
Not enough money	3	2	1	0
Heavy debts	3	2	1	0
Conflicts with mate	3	2	1	0
Conflict over household tasks	3	2	1	0
Problems with children/housemate	3	2	1	0
Pressures from in-laws, family	3	2	1	0
Not enough time with family/friends	3	2	1	0
Work-family conflict	3	2	1	0
Sexual conflict or frustration	3	2	1	0
Dangerous or stressful neighborhood	3	2	1	0
Few friends in neighborhood	3	2	1	0
Time pressures with mate	3	2	1	0

0-4 ○
5-9 ○
10-15 ○
16+ ○

_____ + _____ + _____ + _____ = ○

Scale 5 Total

SCALE 6: Personal Satisfactions

Think of . . . the people closest to you, and your experience with them in the past **month**. *To what degree is each of the following statements true of these relationships?*

	Very	Somewhat	Little	Not At All
The people around me will take time for me when I need it.............................	3	2	1	0
Those closest to me understand when I am upset and respond to me........................	3	2	1	0
I feel accepted and loved by my friends/family ..	3	2	1	0
The people close to me support me to do new things and make changes in my life	3	2	1	0
My mate accepts my sexuality	3	2	1	0
Those closest to me express caring and affection to me	3	2	1	0
I spend high-quality time with friends/family	3	2	1	0
I feel close and in touch with friends/family	3	2	1	0
I am able to give what I would like to my friends/ family..	3	2	1	0
I know that I am important to the people closest to me	3	2	1	0
I am honest with the people close to me and they are honest with me	3	2	1	0
I can ask for help from my family and friends when I need it..............................	3	2	1	0
I can usually find people to "hang out" with	3	2	1	0
I know that others are there for me	3	2	1	0

40 + ○

35-39 ○

27-34 ○

0-26 ○

___ + ___ + ___ + ___ = ○

Scale 6 Total

PART TWO
Coping Responses/Assets and Liabilities

SCALE 7: Self Care

Think about . . . the past **month**. *For each self-care practice, indicate how often each is true for you, or practiced by you.*

	Almost Always	Sometimes	Rarely	Never	
Eat breakfast	3	2	1	0	
Maintain desirable weight	3	2	1	0	
Avoid sugar	3	2	1	0	
Avoid fat	3	2	1	0	
Avoid salt	3	2	1	0	
Do vigorous aerobic exercise	3	2	1	0	
Do stretching or yoga	3	2	1	0	
Enjoy or appreciate my body	3	2	1	0	
Aware of tension in my body when it occurs	3	2	1	0	◯
Brush teeth	3	2	1	0	37+
Fasten seat belts in cars	3	2	1	0	◯
Have a physician I trust who knows me well	3	2	1	0	31-36
Would seek help for an emotional or health problem	3	2	1	0	◯
Relax and take time off	3	2	1	0	22-30
Avoid smoking	3	2	1	0	◯
Avoid excessive alcohol use	3	2	1	0	0-21

_____ + _____ + _____ + _____ = ◯

Scale 7 Total

SCALE 8: Direct Action

Think about . . . the past **month**. *For each statement, indicate to what degree it describes your behavior or intentions.*

	Almost Always	Sometimes	Rarely	Never
I finish what I set out to do	3	2	1	0
I deal with things soon after they come up	3	2	1	0
I find it hard to anticipate difficulties	0	1	2	3
I do as good a job as I can under the circumstances.........................	3	2	1	0
I avoid challenges and new situations	0	1	2	3
I am cautious and shy away from new tasks.....	0	1	2	3
I work to satisfy myself more than others.......	3	2	1	0
I anticipate and plan ahead to meet challenges ..	3	2	1	0
I find it hard to get involved in what I am doing	0	1	2	3
I know how to say "no"	3	2	1	0
I negotiate so that some tasks are more manageable or convenient	3	2	1	0
I do minor tasks to avoid doing major ones	0	1	2	3
When things are difficult I get tired or lose concentration	0	1	2	3

33+ ○
27-32 ○
22-26 ○
0-21 ○

_____ + _____ + _____ + _____ = ○

Scale 8 Total

SCALE 9: Support Seeking

Think about . . . the past **month**. *For each statement, indicate to what degree it describes your behavior or intentions.*

	Almost Always	Sometimes	Rarely	Never
I find someone to work on projects with me	3	2	1	0
I seek information I need from others	3	2	1	0
I try to find someone who can handle a difficult situation...........................	3	2	1	0
I talk over difficult situations with someone I trust	3	2	1	0
I seek advice and support from others..........	3	2	1	0
I am willing to talk about problems with a doctor or counselor	3	2	1	0
I let people know about uncomfortable feelings that are getting in the way of our work	3	2	1	0
I let people know when a task is too much or I am too busy	3	2	1	0

20+ ○
17-19 ○
12-16 ○
0-11 ○

_____ + _____ + _____ + _____ = ○

Scale 9 Total

SCALE 10: Situation Mastery

*Think about . . . the past **month**. For each statement, indicate to what degree it describes your behavior or intentions.*

	Almost Always	Sometimes	Rarely	Never
I am able to take time for myself	3	2	1	0
I find it hard to make time for personal errands ..	0	1	2	3
I eat rapidly and finish meals before other people	0	1	2	3
I get impatient when someone is doing a job that I could do quicker	0	1	2	3
I find time for hobbies or outside interests	3	2	1	0
I hurry even when I have plenty of time	0	1	2	3
I set unrealistic deadlines for myself	0	1	2	3
I push to finish a task, even when I am tired	0	1	2	3
I am hard-driving and competitive	0	1	2	3
Other people set standards for me	0	1	2	3
I'd rather do things myself than get help	0	1	2	3
I find it hard to wait.......................	0	1	2	3
I put other people before myself...............	0	1	2	3
I get great satisfaction from my accomplishments	3	2	1	0

26+
20-25
14-19
0-13

___ + ___ + ___ + ___ = ◯

Scale 10 Total

SCALE 11: Adaptability

*Think about . . . the past **month**. For each statement, indicate to what degree it describes your behavior or intentions.*

	Almost Always	Sometimes	Rarely	Never
I decide certain problems are not worth worrying about	3	2	1	0
I relax myself when tension builds up	3	2	1	0
I can see the humorous side of situations	3	2	1	0
I often put things aside for awhile to get perspective on them	3	2	1	0
I reward myself when I finish a job	3	2	1	0
I put pressures in their place and do not let them overwhelm me	3	2	1	0
I make several alternate plans to deal with situations.................................	3	2	1	0
When I face a problem, I try to get a clear focus on what I could do about it	3	2	1	0

20+
16-19
13-15
0-12

___ + ___ + ___ + ___ = ◯

Scale 11 Total

SCALE 12: Time Management

*Think about . . . the past **month**. For each statement, indicate to what degree it describes your behavior or intentions.*

	Almost Always	Sometimes	Rarely	Never
I use my time efficiently	3	2	1	0
I avoid doing important things.	0	1	2	3
I find it difficult to complete things	0	1	2	3
Distractions keep me from doing what I want . . .	0	1	2	3
People tend to dump tasks on me, and I accept them.	0	1	2	3
I know what I want to be doing	3	2	1	0
I miss appointments or forget important things . .	0	1	2	3
I move from task to task with no reason	0	1	2	3
There is time to accomplish what I expect to do .	3	2	1	0
I do more than I have to on tasks, rather than get on to other things.	0	1	2	3
I am so busy helping others that I don't get my own work done	0	1	2	3

26 +

21-25

16-20

0-15

_____ + _____ + _____ + _____ =

Scale 12 Total

PART THREE

Inner World/Thoughts and Feelings

SCALE 13: Self Esteem

Think about . . . the past **month.** *For each of the following statements, indicate how much each represents the way you think or feel about yourself.*

	Very Much Like Me	Somewhat	Not Very Much	Not At All
I minimize my abilities	3	2	1	0
I wish I were another person	3	2	1	0
I make demands on myself that I would not make on others.	3	2	1	0
I expect others to fault my work	3	2	1	0
I blame myself when things do not work out the way I expect	3	2	1	0
When I succeed I do not think I deserve it	3	2	1	0
I like who I am	0	1	2	3
Under pressure, I think of all the ways things can go wrong	3	2	1	0

0-6 ○
7-10 ○
11-15 ○
16+ ○

____ + ____ + ____ + ____ = ◯

Scale 13 Total

SCALE 14: Positive Outlook

Think about . . . the past **month**. *For each statement, indicate how much each fits the way you think about the world.*

	Very Much	Somewhat	Not Very Much	Not At All
Other people rarely "come through" for me	3	2	1	0
I usually hope for the best	0	1	2	3
I find it hard to look on the bright side of things	3	2	1	0
I am a naturally positive person	0	1	2	3
I have been continually frustrated in my life because of bad breaks.....................	3	2	1	0
The future will probably be better than things are now	0	1	2	3
I seem to get the short end of the stick	3	2	1	0
Very little in life is fair or equitable	3	2	1	0

0-2 ○
3-6 ○
7-10 ○
11+ ○

___ + ___ + ___ + ___ = ○

Scale 14 Total

SCALE 15: Personal Power

Think about . . . the past **month**. *For each statement, indicate how much each is like the way you think or feel about yourself.*

	Very Much Like Me	Somewhat	Not Very Much	Not At All
When things are not going my way, I think it is useless to try to change them	3	2	1	0
My stress seems to be unpredictable	3	2	1	0
I find ways to accomplish what I want.........	0	1	2	3
I am not able to give what I want to people close to me	3	2	1	0
I find myself in situations I feel helpless to do anything about	3	2	1	0
I run into problems I cannot solve	3	2	1	0
I do not think I have control over things in my life	3	2	1	0
I like to take on new challenges	0	1	2	3

0-3 ○
4-7 ○
8-11 ○
12+ ○

___ + ___ + ___ + ___ = ○

Scale 15 Total

SCALE 16: Connection

Think about . . . the past **month**. *For each statement, indicate how much each is like the way you think or feel about yourself.*

	Very Much Like Me	Somewhat	Not Very Much	Not At All	
My work is empty and has no meaning	3	2	1	0	
I feel satisfied with my work	0	1	2	3	
My work feels routine and boring	3	2	1	0	0-3
I feel satisfied with my personal life	0	1	2	3	
Not much is new or unpredictable in my life	3	2	1	0	
My life has a central purpose or goal	0	1	2	3	4-7
My life does not meet my deepest needs	3	2	1	0	
My life is taken up with burdens and responsibilities	3	2	1	0	8-12
I believe there is a higher force or guiding purpose in humanity	0	1	2	3	13 +

_____ + _____ + _____ + _____ = ◯

Scale 16 Total

SCALE 17: Expression

Think about . . . the past **month**. *For each statement, indicate how much each is like the way you think or feel about yourself.*

	Very Much Like Me	Somewhat	Not Very Much	Not At All	
I keep my feelings to myself	3	2	1	0	
I let others know when I am under pressure	0	1	2	3	
I do not like to let people know that I disagree with them	3	2	1	0	0-6
When I am upset, I avoid other people and go off alone	3	2	1	0	7-11
I hold in my anger and frustration	3	2	1	0	
I feel much better when I talk about my feelings	0	1	2	3	
I am afraid of losing control of my feelings	3	2	1	0	12-14
I let others know when I feel angry or disappointed with them	0	1	2	3	15 +

_____ + _____ + _____ + _____ = ◯

Scale 17 Total

SCALE 18: Compassion

Think about . . . the past **month.** *For each statement, indicate how much each is like the way you think or feel about yourself.*

	Very Much Like Me	Somewhat	Not Very Much	Not At All	
When I am upset, I blame someone else for things	3	2	1	0	
I accept other people's differences.............	0	1	2	3	
I blow up with little warning	3	2	1	0	0-2
I feel jealous of others' success	3	2	1	0	
I easily become nasty or irritable	3	2	1	0	3-5
When I feel pressured or frustrated, I fall apart emotionally and lose control	3	2	1	0	6-10
I never know what I will say when I feel angry ..	3	2	1	0	
I make allowances for other people's limitations	0	1	2	3	
I can put myself in other people's shoes	0	1	2	3	11+

_____ + _____ + _____ + _____ = ◯

Scale 18 Total

PART FOUR
Signals of Distress

SCALE 19: Physical Symptoms

*Think about . . . the past **month**. For each of the symptoms listed, indicate how often it has occurred for you.*

	Nearly Every Day	Every Week	Once or Twice	Never	
Muscle tension	3	2	1	0	
Back pain	3	2	1	0	
Headache	3	2	1	0	
Grinding teeth	3	2	1	0	
Stomach ache or upset	3	2	1	0	
Heartburn	3	2	1	0	
Diarrhea	3	2	1	0	○
Constipation	3	2	1	0	0-4
Abdominal pain	3	2	1	0	○
Cold or hay fever	3	2	1	0	5-8
Chest pain	3	2	1	0	○
Shortness of breath	3	2	1	0	9-13
Skin rash	3	2	1	0	○
Dry mouth or sore throat	3	2	1	0	14+
Laryngitis	3	2	1	0	

+ ___ + ___ + ___ = ◯

Scale 19 Total

SCALE 20: Behavioral Symptoms

Think about . . . the past **month**. *Indicate how often you have done or experienced each of the items listed below.*

	Nearly Every Day	Every Week	Once or Twice	Never
Loss of appetite	3	2	1	0
Overeating	3	2	1	0
No time to eat	3	2	1	0
Smoking	3	2	1	0
Drinking alcoholic beverages	3	2	1	0
Taking tranquilizers	3	2	1	0
Taking aspirin and other pain relievers	3	2	1	0
Taking other drugs	3	2	1	0
Withdrawing from close relationships	3	2	1	0
Criticizing, blaming, or ridiculing others	3	2	1	0
Feeling victimized or taken advantage of	3	2	1	0
Watching TV (over 2 hours a day)	3	2	1	0
Overwhelmed by work	3	2	1	0
Difficulty meeting commitments or completing tasks	3	2	1	0
Resent people I encounter at work	3	2	1	0
Hard to pay attention to work tasks	3	2	1	0
Accidents or injuries	3	2	1	0
Distant and uninvolved at work	3	2	1	0

0-7 ◯
8-12 ◯
13-18 ◯
19+ ◯

___ + ___ + ___ + ___ = ◯

Scale 20 Total

SCALE 21: Emotional Symptoms

Think about . . . the past **month**. *For each of the symptoms listed, indicate how often it has occurred.*

	Nearly Every Day	Every Week	Once or Twice	Never
Nervousness or anxiety	3	2	1	0
Tremor or trembling	3	2	1	0
Twitch or tic	3	2	1	0
Keyed-up feeling	3	2	1	0
Cannot turn off certain thoughts	3	2	1	0
Worrying	3	2	1	0
Unable to keep still; fidgeting	3	2	1	0
Irritable; angry emotional outbursts	3	2	1	0
Fatigue	3	2	1	0
Low energy	3	2	1	0
Apathetic; nothing seems important	3	2	1	0
Emotionally drained	3	2	1	0
Loss of sexual interest or pleasure	3	2	1	0
Depressed	3	2	1	0
Fearful	3	2	1	0
Hopeless	3	2	1	0
Crying easily	3	2	1	0
Insomnia	3	2	1	0
Difficulty awakening	3	2	1	0
Too much sleep (over 9 hours)	3	2	1	0
Difficulty concentrating	3	2	1	0
Mind going blank	3	2	1	0
Forgetting important things	3	2	1	0

0-7 ○

8-17 ○

18-29 ○

30 + ○

____ + ____ + ____ + ____ = ○

Scale 21 Total

How to Complete Your StressMap Scoring Grid:

Pull out the Scoring Grid between pages 18 and 19, and lay it flat. (We suggest you make Xerox copies of the Scoring Grid before filling it out, so you will have blank ones for future use.)

The Scoring Grid has four levels for each scale, which correspond to the four scoring levels next to each scale on the Questionnaire. Transfer your scores from the Questionnaire by putting a dot on the corresponding level of the Grid for each of the 21 scales.

Now connect the dots on the Scoring Grid. You'll see they make a zigzag-like pattern. This could be called your "personal stress rhythm." Remember, this pattern represents a "snapshot" of the way you react to stress at a particular moment. It can and probably will change each time you take StressMap, which we suggest doing every three to four months.

Now turn to Section III, The StressMap Interpretation and Action-Planning Guide, for an analysis of what your scores mean, and a discussion of how you can improve your stress hardiness.

III

The StressMap Interpretation and Action-Planning Guide

This section will teach you about your personal performance rhythm, the graph you have plotted on your Scoring Grid. The following pages contain a scale-by-scale interpretation of how you scored on the *StressMap* Questionnaire.

Each interpretation begins with a definition of that scale's area and, when appropriate, a definition of its opposite. This will enable you to see the entire continuum of available positions. The discussion section of each interpretation looks at what you can learn from an analysis of that scale, and it explores the question "Why is this scale important to an understanding of stress in my life?" Finally, we present simple, easy-to-use tips for improving your performance on that scale. These "Tips for Improvement" continue your exploration of stress by involving you in a few guided observations, discoveries, or deductions. These will assist you in becoming clearer about your own motivations and perceptions.

This section of *StressMap* is your personal journal, diary, or log. Record your thoughts and feelings, jot down insights as they occur to you, highlight phrases or sections to which you might want to return. Share it with whomever you wish, or keep it to yourself. Work seriously with it. Pace yourself to make changes one step at a time. Make a month-to-month plan covering a few of the skills you wish to improve in a 12-month period. Use the worksheets and the suggested reading list at the back of the book to help you take action. When you are ready, go on to the next scale you wish to improve.

Do not hesitate to display your Scoring Grid at home or at the office. This visual reminder can reinforce your efforts to make a change or keep an issue in the forefront of your attention. Again, *StressMap* is a snapshot of yourself at the time you took it.

Take *StressMap* again in three months. Essi Systems *StressMap* is a sophisticated device that can measure changes in performance every 12 weeks or so. Use the same Scoring Grid and plot your next graph with a different-colored marker or pen. Compare your different rhythms and map your improvements visually. Monitor your progress. Your *StressMap* will reflect even minor modifications as you strengthen your coping skills, learn to shift your stress attitudes, and develop healthier lifestyle habits. Every time you take the *StressMap* journey, you will have changed.

Understanding Your Personal Stress Rhythm

Essi Systems StressMap will help you chart your performance within four distinct Performance Zones:

Optimal: High level of effectiveness and creativity, even when under pressure.

Balance: Effective and steady performance in most situations.

Strain: Frequent difficulty and sense of feeling overwhelmed or drained.

Burnout: Severe difficulty, impaired functioning, and extreme distress.

The top two zones of the grid, Optimal and Balance, reflect satisfactory performance. A scale whose score falls within one of those zones shows that your effectiveness in that area should be rewarded and maintained. The bottom two zones, Strain and Burnout, reflect degrees of difficulty or distress, and areas in which you score in these zones need your attention.

Now look at your completed Scoring Grid, and observe your stress rhythm. You will probably notice that you have scores in at least three, if not all four, Performance Zones, forming a zigzag graph or pattern.

This pattern is uniquely yours, showing your areas of personal strength and pinpointing your stress "hot spots" or danger areas.

Do you feel disappointed because you scored less than a perfectly straight line in Optimal performance? Would you also feel disappointed if you didn't have a straight line in Burnout? Of course not. We have been taught to want to be perfect. Our definitions of perfection are as flawed as our definitions of peak performance. The keys to stress hardiness are balance and flow. It is more important to achieve a harmonic compatibility among the four major parts of StressMap than it is to excel in any one scale. So view your rhythm as another unique characteristic of who you are.

All of StressMap's 21 scales are based on skills, behaviors, or attitudes that are within your ability to change or modify. If you have more than three Burnouts in one of the four parts of your Scoring Grid, be alert to the potential health risks you are exposing yourself to and immediately take steps to change these attitudes and behaviors. You should seek out medical or other health-care professionals if you are experiencing any physical, emotional, or behavioral deterioration or breakdown of any kind. Bring your StressMap with you.

Part One:
Your Environment/Pressures and Satisfactions

Part One: Your Environment/Pressures and Satisfactions has six scales that explore both your personal world of family, spouse, and friends and your work world of job, company, and colleagues. In each you experience changes and pressures as well as support and satisfactions. Part One measures external stress factors—circumstances and activities that are currently affecting you. Changes in your personal world demand energy and attention that may distract you at work or in other parts of your life. Changes in your work world, and daily work and personal stresses, require adaptation and can strongly influence your sense of personal value and your ability to control life events.

Satisfactions act to offset pressures and changes, often balancing, sometimes supporting, the rest of that part. If you are unable to decrease the pressures in your environment, you may find that you can increase the satisfactions to balance them.

Let's look at Maria Perez's Scoring Grid. Maria is a 37-year-old bank manager, and she supervises more than 11 employees. She has been at this particular job for two years, and has been with the bank for more than eight years.

In the past year, Maria has had few Work Changes, so there is high stability in her work setting and areas of responsibility. She is, however, experiencing Strain as a result of Work Pressures. Her Balanced performance on Work Satisfactions may help her manage these pressures.

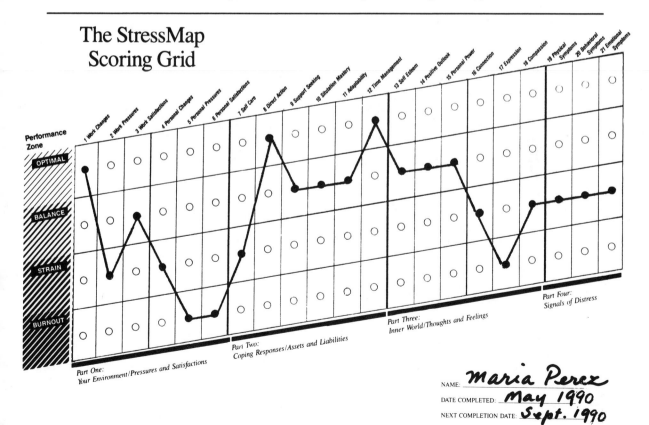

The StressMap Scoring Grid

Performance Zone: OPTIMAL, BALANCE, STRAIN, BURNOUT

1 Work Changes, 2 Work Pressures, 3 Work Satisfactions, 4 Personal Changes, 5 Personal Pressures, 6 Personal Satisfactions, 7 Self Care, 8 Direct Action, 9 Support Seeking, 10 Situation Mastery, 11 Adaptability, 12 Time Management, 13 Self Esteem, 14 Positive Outlook, 15 Personal Power, 16 Connection, 17 Expression, 18 Compassion, 19 Physical Symptoms, 20 Behavioral Symptoms, 21 Emotional Symptoms

Part One: Your Environment/Pressures and Satisfactions

Part Two: Coping Responses/Assets and Liabilities

Part Three: Inner World/Thoughts and Feelings

Part Four: Signals of Distress

NAME: *Maria Perez*
DATE COMPLETED: *May 1990*
NEXT COMPLETION DATE: *Sept. 1990*

It is more likely that her Work Satisfactions and her stability on Work Changes are offsetting the disturbing state of her personal world right now. Maria's ratings show Burnout in both Personal Pressures and Personal Satisfactions and Strain in Personal Changes. She may be undergoing a great deal of chaos and transition in her life, such as a divorce or problems with household members. The demands placed on her both emotionally and physically can be seen in her Strain ratings in all three Signals of Distress, Scales 19, 20, and 21. These indicate a rather high level of wear and tear on her physical and emotional health.

Maria needs to move one or two of her Burnouts into Strain or one of her Strains into Balance. If she tries to increase her Personal Satisfactions, more Personal Changes might be required, placing her under even greater stress.

Maria would be wise to ask herself which of the Coping Responses scales, or the Inner World scales, she thinks is most connected to her Signals of Distress. How can she begin her renewal?

Maria scored low on Self Care, Physical Symptoms, and Emotional Symptoms. It is very important that she find some kind of physical release, such as exercise, and some form of emotional release, such as speaking to a counselor or sharing her feelings with someone she trusts. Maria could take advantage of her skill in Support Seeking and perhaps ask for assistance in locating resources to help her relieve some of her Personal Pressures.

Now look at your own Scoring Grid, and jot down any links between Your Environment and other *StressMap* scales that you think might be connected. (Space for jotting down personal notes is provided at the end of each Part of this Interpretation section.) Write down why they might be related, and then read the following scale-by-scale interpretation.

SCALE 1: Work Changes

Definition

Work Changes are on-the-job events that represent a shift or variation from something usual or constant to something new or different, such as relocation or a new project. These event-initiated changes, which are discussed in the section "Coping With a Changing World," are marked by the substitution of one set of circumstances for another and demand a period of transition.

Discussion

All change, positive or negative, chosen or unchosen, requires that you make some adjustments. You may need to deal with newness and the unknown; find yourself coping with feelings of uncertainty and self-doubt; experience the grief that frequently accompanies change, since with every beginning there is an ending; or feel overwhelmed.

In times of change, the magnitude of what you are experiencing may at times seem like more than you can handle. The enormity of your feelings has its source both in the disruption of the patterns in your daily life and in some level of self-examination that inevitably accompanies change. This process is what makes change hard.

Regardless of the results that changes bring or your personal reactions to them, all change demands energy and attention. Your body must be prepared to respond because, unlike mechanical equipment, the human system requires more than the flick of a switch or the turning of a few knobs to adjust itself.

Tips for Improvement

• **Temporarily alter your routine to accommodate change.** It is very difficult to manage all the newness that change brings while maintaining a full work schedule and personal life. Temporarily accommodate these special demands by hiring extra office or household help. If that is not an option, don't be afraid to ask friends or colleagues for support. Acknowledge to yourself that you *do* need help during this time.

• **Safeguard your health above all.** To offset the physical and psychic drains of high-stress times, replenish yourself with much-needed periods of rest and renewal, exercise, a healthy low-fat diet, and leisure time with friends and family. Build in mini-R&R breaks like hot baths, time away from your desk, lunchtime visits with friends, or weekend escapes.

• **Express both your fear and excitement about the change.** Sometimes we focus only on the excitement of change, suppressing fears or doubts we may have because we don't want to feel vulnerable or weak. However, these denied emotions tend to find their expression in our bodies as illness. When the crisis passes or the "main event" of the change is over, our unexpressed fears may show themselves as colds, sore throats, fatigue, rashes or other forms of sickness.

• **Keep changes in perspective.** Remember that transition is the process of adjustment after a change has occurred. You must become familiar with your new environment before you can feel confident and productive again.

• **Limit crisis orientation as much as possible.** Most of us love a crisis—the flurry of activity and the need for quick decision-making are exciting. While most crises are not life-threatening, we act as though they are. In time, such behavior can become addictive, which may interfere with clear thinking in times of change and may cause damage to our health. A state of chronic red alert is physically exhausting.

Definition

Work Pressures are those on-the-job relationships, situations, or issues that you perceive as constraining, difficult, or draining. Pressures are ongoing influences and are not marked by a shift or event, as Work Changes are.

Discussion

Work Pressures are the daily hassles of work life. Some pressures are easy to identify, such as a difficult commute or the steady drone of loud machinery or equipment. Other pressures are more subtle and relentless, like the hum of fluorescent lighting, dealing with difficult co-workers, or the tension of office politics.

Everyone responds differently to these pressures. Often you don't notice the toll they extract until your headache is in full throb or your neck is tight from tension. Effective stress management requires that you learn to cope with different pressures in distinct ways. Handling interpersonal issues may involve a different coping strategy than would problems with your job performance or conflict with some organizational policy, and it may also require greater communications skills.

Not all pressure is bad. Meeting deadlines and demands can feel exhilarating and may contribute to a sense of competence and creativity. Time expectations, when realistically considered, can motivate activity and help structure tasks.

Not liking your job, or feeling little dedication to your work, are passive pressures that eventually will sap your spirit and your productivity. Identify what you can or cannot change about the pressures you feel, and try to find some aspect of every pressure that you *can* respond to.

Tips for Improvement

● **Notice tension in your body and use stress-release techniques.** Notice tension in your body when you are under pressure. This is a signal that can alert you to stress build-up. Deep sighs, tight neck and shoulder muscles, stomach cramps or aches, fatigue—all may be signals of distress. As soon as you notice any of these symptoms, stop what you are doing and take a few deep breaths. (It is physiologically impossible to maintain the same level of body tension before and after a deep breath.)

● **Identify the Work Pressures you perceive as most stressful.** Everyone has an area of pressure that is more draining than others. Some of you may resent your work as boring or unrewarding. Others may fear conflict with co-workers, suffer confusion about job expectations, or dread performance reviews. Identifying your most severe area of pressure is the first step to understanding how to ease it.

● **Take steps to alleviate pressures you *can* do something about.** Learn to find some part of the pressure that you can respond to and take action. For example, if your boss is placing too many demands on you, while you might not be able to change his or her behavior, you *can* establish limits and priorities that are personally manageable for you, such as leaving the office on time, setting realistic deadlines, and having a clear sense of expectations.

● **Create a "safety valve" for dealing with emergency-level pressures.** Many people find it helpful to have a contingency plan for times that seem utterly overwhelming. Plan for such times and prepare a course of alternative action for personal mental health. Think of a phrase to help you put pressures in perspective, or close your eyes and imagine a time when you felt peaceful and calm. Use quick calming techniques to prevent the build-up of inner distress.

Definition

Work Satisfactions are those on-the-job relationships, situations, or issues that you perceive as fulfilling or desirable. In the Optimal position you find many positive benefits that bring enjoyment and challenge into your day-to-day work experience. The Burnout position reflects extreme job frustration.

Discussion

The Work Satisfactions scale is the opposite of the Work Pressures scale; the two complement each other. Each of us views work through his or her own set of expectations. Many of us are able to overlook, or at least not dwell on, Work Pressures by consciously choosing to emphasize our Work Satisfactions.

Feeling valued, receiving adequate compensation, and using talents and abilities on the job all contribute to our level of work satisfaction. Every individual has a set of personal expectations or needs that make the effort of getting up and going to work worthwhile.

If you think of yourself as being in a relationship with your work, you can examine how you interact within this relationship. What do you like most about it? Do you wake up each day and look forward to doing the work you choose? Knowing what you value most in life will help you find and re-create it on the job, so that your work becomes a constant source of renewal and excitement.

Many employees think that every job is fixed, with a rigid set of definitions and conditions and no allowance for idiosyncrasies. In most cases, though, a job is only what you bring to it. Every day you are involved in an active process of deciding, choosing, interacting, making requests, undertaking tasks, negotiating, working with others,

questioning, and planning how to accomplish your projects. The person defines the job, not vice versa. If you find little opportunity for self expression in your job or work, the gap between what you want and what the job demands may warrant a new job search.

Tips for Improvement

● **Identify elements of your job that you presently enjoy.** Write down as many satisfactions or things you enjoy about your present job as you can. (Push yourself to list at least 10.) Then go back and put a "P" next to those that are people-related. ("I like my boss." "We have a good team." "Barbara has become my best friend." "I like to play cards during lunch.")

Put an "S" next to those that are related to your own skills or abilities. ("I can be creative." "I like to figure things out." "I get to use my hands." "The work is manageable." "I get to make decisions." "I'm always learning new things.")

Lastly, put a "J" next to those satisfactions that are related to the job. (The physical work environment. Your salary or wage. Being outdoors. Good benefits. Close to home. Convenient hours. Good child care. Opportunity for advancement.)

Now examine your list to see whether you have many more of one letter than others. Try to balance these areas of satisfaction by working on the ones that now seem to be giving you less satisfaction.

● **Find ways to turn frustrations into satisfactions.** Most of us are not clear about what will make us feel satisfied. One way to find out is to take the opposite and turn it around. Ask yourself what your major frustration is. Then look at its opposite. If it is boredom or lack of opportunity, ask yourself what would offer excitement or advancement. Seek to create it in this job.

SCALE **4: Personal Changes**

Definition

Personal Changes are events in your personal world of mate, family, and friends that represent a shift from something usual or constant to something new or different. These changes can be represented by an event, a decision, an issue, or a person.

Discussion

Your mate, family, and close friends comprise your inner circle. Within this circle you establish patterns of interacting and behaving and develop a style or pattern of relating that is based on your personal needs, expectations, goals, and values.

When a major event, positive or negative, alters or disrupts your usual style, the change may be difficult for you. As with Work Changes, Personal Changes require adjustment or adaptation to make the unknown familiar. An illness or injury is rarely anticipated and will require a definite period of adjustment. It may often be accompanied by grief or frustration. Anyone who has ever experienced loss due to death, divorce, or distance has surely felt out of step with his or her usual style.

Personal Changes, like the decision to be clean and sober, to enter therapy, or to quit smoking, will all require transition adjustments, and, in some cases, life-long shifts. Personal Changes are far-reaching and long-lasting. Changes caused by an injury, an accident, or an assault can have a profound effect on the individual and his or her circle. You cannot always prepare for some of these changes.

An observation made during research on Essi Systems *StressMap* suggests that Personal Changes are experienced as more stressful than comparable Work Changes. Many employees reported that Personal Changes, losses, and transitions were far more difficult to manage and cope with than Work Changes. Many of us look to our inner circle of spouse, family, and friends for support and love, and can feel shattered if we do not find it there.

Tips for Improvement

● **Be gentle and patient with yourself when making or going through Personal Changes.** Abandon thoughts based on "shoulds"—"I should be used to this by now," "I should have reached my goal yesterday." If the Personal Change you are experiencing is one you have chosen, imagine yourself as having successfully made the change: being a nonsmoker, being a happy person, working in a new career. If possible, be specific with your images and enjoy this vision of the new you.

Sometimes Personal Changes—for example, losses—are not of our own choosing and are beyond our immediate control. If these occur, give yourself time and loving care during the period of adaptation to the change. If you need it, seek professional help. Support yourself with a circle of friends who know and love you.

● **Let go of things outside your control.** Don't "overcontrol" as a way of dealing with stressful and unfamiliar situations. Allow for vulnerable times of confusion and grief. You can't control the traffic, the weather, your children, or your boss. But you *can* control your reactions to them.

● **Avoid negative "quick fixes."** Be careful not to "reward" yourself in ways that actually place more stress on your body. Drinking more alcohol than usual, using drugs, smoking cigarettes, overeating, or indulging in too much of anything are attempts to feel good that have negative consequences.

SCALE **5**: **Personal Pressures**

Definition

Personal Pressures are ongoing relationships, situations, and issues in your personal and family worlds that you perceive as constraining, difficult, or draining. Pressures are the everyday events to which you must respond emotionally and physically. In the Optimal position, pressures are manageable with minimal personal distress.

Discussion

Every day you make decisions and tend to the needs and wants of those in your personal and family worlds. Conflicts with your mate, household tasks, time issues, or worry about money can become chronic or unmanageable pressures that mount up to pose serious health problems.

Running a household today is much like performing a juggling act—the needs of children, career, spouse, elderly parents, and close friends can make it hard for you to find time to take care of yourself. Yet your own needs demand continued attention and require active decision making, with a clear sense of priorities. Chronic stress build-up from relentless Personal Pressures diminishes mental alertness, stifles creativity, and dulls sexual interest and performance. The more unmanageable these pressures feel, the greater the need for relief. Often negative "quick fixes," such as excessive drinking, drug use, binge spending, binge eating, and so on, provide a superficial sense of release, which actually contributes only to increased demands on the body.

Tips for Improvement

• **Avoid destructive or cloaking behaviors that offer short-term solutions to long-term problems.** Drinking, drugs, and violent behavior are short-term indulgences that inhibit your ability to deal with long-term problems. Replace negative fixes with positive ones: Make plans to get together with close friends or relatives after dinner; avoid the temptation to withdraw from or neglect social needs.

• **Offset pressures with time for quiet relaxation and activities that bring you pleasure.** Engage in any form of personal expression that will help you keep ongoing pressures in perspective. Take time every day to rest and be quiet. Turn off any negative self-talk and clear your mind by focusing on your breathing or heart rate.

• **Go into therapy and/or join a support group.** Personal pressures can often seem overwhelming. When this happens, we sometimes need professional help to guide us through difficult times.

• **Shift your perspective to discover new options.** Often we can't see beyond our daily pressures to find a way to change our circumstances. Look at your Personal Pressures questionnaire for Scale 5 and select an item that is a source of great pressure for you. If "not enough time with family and friends" is a problem, imagine what actually having enough time would be like. What one thing can you do to change this? Take a chance and act on it!

• **Listen to and follow your feelings about your life.** They'll give you an honest response to what's going on. Many times we rationalize putting up with a situation that we are actually capable of changing. If you are in a difficult situation that cannot be changed, reexamine your attitude toward it. If possible, view it as a chance to learn or an opportunity for growth.

SCALE 6: **Personal Satisfactions**

Definition

Personal Satisfactions are the ongoing relationships, situations, and issues in your personal world that bring joy, pleasure, and contentment. These strongly contribute to your sense of well-being and add to your vitality and zest for life. In the Burnout position, this scale measures extreme frustration with existing support systems and opportunities for growth.

Discussion

Satisfactions in your personal world are derived from connections with those closest to you and contribute to your sense of belonging. They offer an endless supply of intangibles that feel fulfilling and rewarding, like playing with children, pulling together in tough times, getting together with friends for the holidays, and knowing that others will be there for you when you need them.

Satisfactions can also derive from opportunities for personal growth and development. Expressing yourself creatively, making new friends, having adventures, learning new skills, or experiencing different cultures can all infuse you with excitement and energy, requiring you to refresh or renew talents and abilities. Satisfactions serve to revitalize your spirit and increase your sense of challenge and self worth.

The highest levels of stress problems exist when Personal Pressures far outweigh Personal Satisfactions. The burden of day-to-day management of household and relationship issues without the balance of Personal Satisfactions creates feelings of helplessness and futility, and can result in strain, conflict, and poor self esteem.

Tips for Improvement

● **Reach beyond your last known limit.** In sports, an athlete finds great satisfaction in exceeding his or her own personal best. You can derive pleasure from actively working toward new goals. Push yourself to set limits that feel challenging and require a disciplined, dedicated effort to achieve.

● **Take up a new hobby, learn a new skill, or work toward some goal you've been saying you want to attain.** Bring satisfaction into your life by creating opportunities for new experiences. Make a list of all the things you say you want to do, or wish you had more time for. Ask yourself what keeps you from doing these things. Explore the ways you keep yourself stuck in a rut or frustrated. Pick one hobby, skill, or goal and use the Action-Planning Worksheet in the back of this book to help you master it.

● **Seek to eliminate Burnout factors, and strengthen meaningful relationships.** If you find that the people closest to you are not there for you when you need them, that they are not providing the support and encouragement you need to try new things, or that frustrations are blocking your efforts to grow, you must begin immediately to find the resources to change this. Take a close look at how you're trying to create satisfactions. Do you clearly and directly ask others for what you want or need? Do you give the kind of support that you expect from others? Do you use lack of support from others to keep you from making decisions for yourself? Try taking the first step. Be honest about your feelings and about asking for help when you need it.

YOUR PERSONAL NOTES ON PART ONE

*Date:*_____

_____

_____

_____

_____

_____

_____

_____

*Date:*_____

_____

_____

_____

_____

_____

_____

_____

*Date:*_____

_____

_____

_____

_____

_____

_____

_____

YOUR PERSONAL NOTES ON PART ONE

Date: _____

_____

_____

_____

_____

_____

_____

_____

Date: _____

_____

_____

_____

_____

_____

_____

_____

Date: _____

_____

_____

_____

_____

_____

_____

_____

Part Two: Coping Responses/Assets and Liabilities

Part Two: Coping Responses/Assets and Liabilities deals with the ways you act in stressful situations. Part Two helps you explore some of the characteristic ways you learned to deal with stress from your experience, your education, and your upbringing.

Many of us learn how to respond to crisis situations and stressful conditions by example. Adult members of the household in which you were raised may be the role models you learned from, and the ones you still use. *StressMap* will help you assess the relative strength of your coping style in each of six scales that measure qualities considered essential to effective stress management. If your score falls in the Strain or Burnout zone, the skills you learned may need to be updated, or modified. If your scores range in the Balance or Optimal zone, you may want to reinforce what you are doing well.

Michael Baxter is a 33-year-old operations manager at a New York brokerage house. He has been divorced for two years and lives alone. Mike's profile shows that some of his coping skills are well developed and some aren't. Within Part Two, Mike has one Burnout, the lowest possible zone, and one Optimal, the highest possible zone. Let's look at these two zones. Time Management is Mike's strongest suit. He sets priorities and weights decisions extremely efficiently. Direct Action, the ability to meet challenges head on, is Mike's area of least proficiency.

Mike has three important coping skills that serve him well. Self Care, Scale 7, shows positive lifestyle habits; Support Seeking, Scale 9, affirms his ability to ask others for help when he needs it; and Time Management, Scale 12, shows his excellent use of time to get things done.

Mike's scores on Adaptability and Sit-

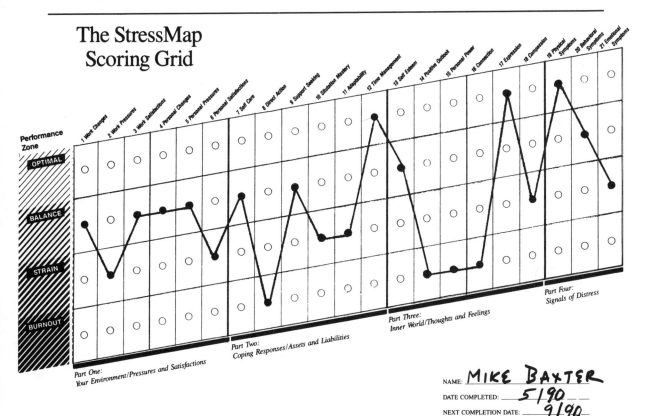

The StressMap Scoring Grid

NAME: MIKE BAXTER
DATE COMPLETED: 5/90
NEXT COMPLETION DATE: 9/90

uation Mastery show that he may be reacting inappropriately to some situation or event beyond his control, and that he may be unable to shift from his usual way of approaching some pressure in his life. Work Pressures are causing a Strain position in Part One, and he may feel frustrated with his lack of Personal Satisfactions. Despite poor coping in some areas, Mike has balanced some of his Strain with good coping skills in others.

Notice Scales 19, 20, and 21, the Signals of Distress. He has one Optimal, one Balance, and one Strain. His coping skills in Part Two are connected to his scores in Part Four. Can you think of how they might be related?

Look at your own Scoring Grid, and make any notes you wish to come back to. Read the following interpretations of Coping Responses/Assets and Liabilities, and explore the meaning of your scores.

SCALE 7: Self Care

Definition

Self Care comprises regular habits of taking care of your body; it includes nutrition, exercise, rest, and hygiene. Self Care reflects how you meet your physical needs and is an expression of your self esteem. The opposite position on this scale is self neglect, or disregard for your personal well-being.

Discussion

Self Care shows how effectively you care for your body when you are under stress. Your attentiveness to the conditions and needs of your physical self can strengthen your immune system, improve your productivity and humor, and bolster your body's regenerative qualities.

Body awareness, fitness, and self maintenance are major components of high performance, and they must be worked into your daily routine if you are to perform optimally. A healthy body has the resilience to bounce back from daily pressures, and it can bring you pleasure and enjoyment as well.

More than the simple mechanics of caring for your body's needs, Self Care shows that you value yourself. Making the time and taking the energy to pamper yourself or give yourself everything you need for good health are important for your emotional as well as physical well-being. Even brushing your teeth twice a day demonstrates Self Care.

Many self-care practices are prevention-oriented and act to delay or minimize the effects of the physical wear and tear of stress. Avoiding sugars and fats may not appear necessary for a healthy 20-year-old, yet the awareness and practice of lowering fat intake will be appreciated by this 20-year-old in 20 years. A person who practices positive health habits can increase his or her life expectancy by up to 5 years.*

Tips for Improvement

• **Make small changes, one at a time.** Go back to your *StressMap* Questionnaire, and select one and only one practice that you rarely or never follow. You don't have to select the most difficult or most neglected area; pick one you think you can actually change. Be realistic about the desired goal. For example, if you don't regularly eat breakfast, begin doing so twice a week. Use the Action-Planning Worksheet in the book to help you plan for this change. As with any new resolution, if you haven't made plans for change, you probably won't change.

• **Do not abuse alcohol or drugs. Do not smoke.** If you smoke or drink excessively, or misuse or abuse any substance, stop. Substance abuse and dependency are serious threats to your physical, emotional, and spiritual well-being. Whether cigarettes, alcohol, marijuana, cocaine, or another drug, if it creates problems, then it is a problem. Seek professional assistance or join an AA-type support group to help you explore the nature and cause of your abuse.

• **Develop healthy eating patterns.** Balance is the key to a healthy diet. Supplying your body with its daily minimum requirements of minerals, vitamins, and other nutrients keeps all of its systems in sync and allows for well-tuned physical, mental, and emotional functioning.

• **Develop a regular weekly exercise plan.** At least three times a week, the body needs to tone its muscles, cleanse its system of residual toxins that build up in the blood-

---

* *Almeda County Health and Ways of Living Study*, 1968–1978.

stream, and release stress tensions. This can be accomplished through aerobic exercise sustained for a specified amount of time to allow exertion. Regular exercise increases your energy levels, keeps your appetite in check, strengthens your physical endurance, and uses up stored fats. Walking, swimming, running, jogging, sustained aerobic dancing, stretching, playing basketball, and racquetball or any other racquet sport require use of the large muscles. Large-muscle exercises are primarily responsible for dissipation of body fat.

SCALE **8**: Direct Action

Definition

Direct Action is the ability to face demands head-on, complete achievable tasks, and reach goals with little distraction. As stressors arise, the skilled direct action taker feels confident of his or her ability to respond satisfactorily. Optimal performers on this scale make decisions and take actions consistent with their personal priorities, goals, and values. They know what they can and cannot achieve. The opposite of Direct Action is avoidance, the tendency to procrastinate or postpone completion of a goal, task, or purpose.

Discussion

Direct Action involves knowing what your priorities are, what you value, and whether or not you can successfully complete what you set out to do. Both this scale and the Adaptability scale address your ability to shift gears, assess the appropriate action to take, and allot the time and energy needed to deal with problems by rearranging tasks and priorities. Making some tasks more manageable, setting realistic timetables for getting things done, being *proactive* in planning rather than *reactive,* and dealing with things as soon as they come up are all examples of high-performance behaviors on this scale.

Research suggests avoidance practices can stem from several sources. Procrastination has been linked to perfectionism, as well as fear of success or failure. Such fear or lack of faith in yourself can lead you to avoid action completely.

In addition, taking direct action or avoiding it is a learned behavior that you develop as a way of dealing with difficult or unknown situations. You may need to examine and modify these patterns of behav-ior if you find yourself in the Strain or Burnout zones of this scale. A score of 26 or lower would indicate a need for you to learn new Direct Action skills.

Tips for Improvement

• **Finish what you set out to do.** One major Direct Action skill is the ability to finish what you start. Follow through. If you continually have difficulty completing projects, you might be taking on tasks that are too large. Or you may lack perseverance because of wavering dedication. Or you may be unable to ask for help when you need it. Before you start, choose goals that are achievable, plan realistically, and reward yourself for meeting short-term deadlines.

• **Concentrate on the most important tasks first.** If you spend a great deal of time on minor tasks, you may be avoiding major ones. Ask yourself why you shy away from tasks that would mean the most to you. Fear or anxiety may sabotage your efforts to move ahead or accept new challenges.

• **Take inventory of your present skills or levels of proficiency.** Sometimes we procrastinate because we lack necessary skills. Assess your needs and learn the basic competencies. If you procrastinate, even with the prerequisite skills behind you, then the issue may be more one of motivation than ability.

• **Work to please yourself.** When you value the work you do because you believe in it, or think it important, then your work tends to be easier to do. Focus on some aspect or result of your work that satisfies you, and keep that image in mind as you work.

• **Examine beliefs that may limit the work you do.** Jobs that are perceived as busy work, menial, or unimportant are often cited as major causes of avoidance. They hold no excitement or value for us. Of course, we all have to do some types of work that are less exciting than others, but if you spend the majority of your time this way, you might consider why you keep yourself in limiting work that poses no challenges. Even people who acknowledge that they seek more stimulation report that at least some aspects of their work are worthwhile.

SCALE 9: Support Seeking

Definition

Support Seeking is the ability to ask others for help when you need it and to share with them your needs, thoughts, and feelings. Support can take the form of knowledge, physical or financial assistance, or emotional caring. The opposite of Support Seeking is withdrawal, moving away from others, being unwilling to communicate needs, or refusing help when it is offered.

Discussion

Think of this scale as your resource or support directory. The more capable you are of creating and using networks of friends, colleagues, and advisers, the more information and assistance—and ultimately power—you can gain with a call or visit. When faced with new or first-time experiences (like buying your first home, starting a business, taking a class, or speaking in front of a group) or when coping with difficult situations or issues (like caring for elderly parents, raising children, dealing with the prejudices of others, or thinking about divorce), Support Seeking provides two invaluable opportunities.

First, you will have an advisory panel of sorts through whom you can learn to avoid mistakes, hear what to expect, explore alternatives, and get advice on legal, financial, banking, tax, and other technical matters, which are often a source of stress. Second, a circle of support, whether it is large or small, can act as an emotional safety net. Knowing that someone will be there during times of imbalance and stress, whether you choose to use that safety net or not, can enhance your sense of personal power and self-confidence. Not surprisingly, people who ask for and receive help and support from others also seem able to offer help to others when needed.

Tips for Improvement

● **Ask for help when you need it.** When overwhelmed with Personal or Work Pressures, seek the information or assistance you need from others. If you think needing help is a sign of weakness, or feel too embarrassed, confused, or fearful of others' judgments, practice Support Seeking by picking one thing you wish to request. Prepare yourself, and ask someone whom you are reasonably certain can provide what you want and is willing to give it to you.

● **Learn to seek support from yourself as well as from others.** Is there such a thing as too much Support Seeking? Yes. Overreliance on the advice, actions, opinions, or judgments of others can lead to feeling helpless yourself. Learn to listen to your intuition, and trust your own experience in making wise decisions.

● **Create wide support nets.** Make a list of your areas of need. Who do you seek out for your social and friendship needs, business and career needs, personal and family needs, spiritual and emotional needs, financial and legal needs, political and community needs, and medical and health-care needs? Ask friends to recommend good lawyers, doctors, schools, and so on, and then use your own judgment to make final decisions.

SCALE **10**: Situation Mastery

Definition

Situation Mastery is the balancing of and coping with situations and events so that you don't overreact, underreact, or react inappropriately. The Optimal position reflects a high capacity to take action when you are in control and to recognize when situations are beyond your control. The Burnout position on this scale could be called "ceaseless striving," or the endless struggle to control the uncontrollable.

Discussion

Being constantly competitive, trying to change someone's character, setting unrealistic deadlines—all of these are signs of poor Situation Mastery. Any one of these behaviors by itself would not be cause for concern, and certainly any ambitious individual might take pride in his or her personal determination. However, when one is relentlessly pushing, demanding, or hurrying, even when there is no real need to do so, the behavior is inappropriate. It places undue strains on the body. If you've ever tried to change a spouse's behavior, or a teenager's bad habit, then you know how futile it can be to try to control the uncontrollable.

This scale deals with the delicate balance of choosing behaviors and responses that are appropriate to the situation. Knowing how and when to push ahead or back off, to assert or accept, to drive or coast, is important for a healthy balancing between too much and too little pressure. The key skills of Situation Mastery are patience, prioritizing, pacing, and setting reasonable expectations.

Tips for Improvement

● **Assess your "ceaseless striving" re-** sponses. Become aware of times when you overreact, respond with undue anger or resentment, or disregard important personal wants or obligations. Resentments or hostilities associated with competition, or perfectionistic approaches to tasks, can impair your physical well-being.

● **Respond to the part of every situation that you can control.** When you find that you feel impatient, irritated, upset, or anxious, ask yourself, "What do I need right now that would make me feel better?" Answer this with something that you can control. Instead of some statement like, "I need my boss to be on time," say, "I am not going to waste my time waiting for my boss to be on time." Look for some way to use the time that will benefit you. Sit quietly, call a friend, or do something else that will save you time later. In this way, you release stress and master situations that might otherwise hinder your performance and leave you feeling angry.

● **Reduce your sense of urgency.** Learn to take deep breaths instead of cursing at the driver in front of you who is going too slowly. Sing, hum, or distract yourself when stuck in traffic. Plan for times when you know you generally feel impatient, like waiting for lines to move or meetings to start. Visualizations are quick, easy mental exercises that reduce stress build-up. Imagine a pleasant scene or memory when you feel that urgency or impatience is getting the best of you.

● **Use time-management skills to prioritize tasks and goals.** Finally, your mastery of situations will be greatly improved if you use good time-management skills. Be realistic and allow enough time for the completion of tasks and appointments.

SCALE 11: Adaptability

Definition

Adaptability is the ability to shift gears, change directions, take time off, and try different strategies to manage difficult situations. Optimal performers demonstrate remarkable flexibility in coping with challenges and demands. The Burnout position on this scale reflects rigidity, inflexibility, or unwillingness to shift from automatic reactions that don't work to more effective, though less familiar, responses.

Discussion

Like Direct Action and Situation Mastery, Adaptability requires the skill of balancing. The Adaptability scale measures your willingness to experiment with new strategies and new approaches to solving problems, risking the familiar for the chance for more reward.

Adaptability skills enable wise decision making. You can cause great inner distress when you rely on only a few characteristic ways of responding to difficult situations, particularly when none of them worked very well the last time. High performers here keep pressures in perspective by having a contingency plan to fall back on and cultivating a sense of humor that can be called on to break up tensions when appropriate.

Adaptability is particularly important during times of change. For example, if your company is part of a merger, you may need to adjust to a new boss, a modified set of goals for your division, or new co-workers. You may even be asked to relocate. You'll be most successful during such changes by remaining flexible, resilient, and capable of adapting to new information and circumstance.

Tips for Improvement

● **Step back and examine a situation before responding.** Attempt to put pressures in their place and not let them overwhelm you. Stop before you respond in a rigid, habitual way. Detach yourself momentarily to consider options, and then try one. Avoid the temptation to slip into familiar old responses that aren't very effective for you.

● **Examine obstacles to personal success.** Think about a situation in which you were trying out a new strategy or behavior. What was most difficult for you? How did you feel? New ways of behaving feel awkward and unnatural when you first attempt them. Unless there is some strong motivation and reinforcement for staying with it, going back to your old familiar ways is much simpler. Use the Action-Planning Worksheet to target specific reinforcements for sticking with new behaviors.

● **Identify personal patterns of rigid coping, and turn one around.** You may want to identify patterns of rigidity that you would like to alter. To do this, observe yourself for one day. Note how you react to compliments, to demands, to angry co-workers. Maybe you're rigid only when it comes to dealing with your boss or your children. How many of your reactions were automatic or programmed? Pick a "rehearsed response" that you wish to change, and develop a plan to shift that behavior to be more spontaneous. Identify the hardest habits to break.

● **Get coaching or outside help in shifting deeply ingrained behaviors.** You may need to get some help when trying to alter long-standing behaviors. Asking someone to monitor and assist you in changing this behavior will give you support and feedback on your progress.

SCALE **12**: Time Management

Definition

Time Management is the use of time as an essential resource through which tasks and activities are arranged, based on your priorities and the demands others place on you. The opposite of Time Management is disorganization, which leads to chaos and a cycle of stressful habits.

Discussion

When the day is in full swing, you can get caught up in the demands of the moment. If your work or personal goals are not clearly ordered, daily pressures will cause "tunnel vision" and distract you from overall objectives. Managing your time is therefore an effective stress-management practice.

Sometimes disorganization is a way to avoid power or success. If you find that you focus on minor tasks and activities instead of doing important things, you may want to ask yourself why. There are hundreds of things that could occupy your time. If we were to judge your priorities based on how you spend your time, what could we say about you? Think about your usual work day and the amount of time you spend on various tasks like writing memos, going to meetings, or inspecting production lines. Rate these tasks A, B, or C, according to their importance to you. When push comes to shove, do you instantly know how to get the A's done, the B's delegated, and the C's reshuffled or discarded?

Tips for Improvement

• **List three of your major personal and professional life goals.** Write down three of your major personal and professional life goals. How do you want to achieve these? Goals can act as yardsticks against which activities and tasks can be measured. When an activity comes up, you can ask yourself, "Does this take me closer to or farther from my goal—is this an A, B, or C task?" If it brings you closer, you probably consider it important. If it doesn't bring you closer, or if it takes you farther away, you should defer it or leave it undone. Try to spend most of your quality time on the A tasks.

• **Find a time-planning system that helps you.** Use some time-management system that can work for you on a day-to-day basis. There are many different types of calendar and planning systems on the market. Some help you to manage time, goals, and projects and include space for recording expenses, notes, and other key information. Some are more simple. Experiment with different kinds until you find the one that works for you. Feel free to devise your own.

• **Organize a work space that fits your needs.** Set up a work space that suits your needs and minimizes distractions. Proper lighting and ventilation, easy access to materials, and pleasant posters are some of the things that enhance our ability to focus on the work or task to be done and not the space it is being done in.

• **Set realistic time boundaries, and communicate them to others.** Find a way to let others know that you are focusing your attention on an important task. If you do not wish to be interrupted during the hours you make sales phone calls, you can post a sign or symbol on the door that alerts your colleagues to your schedule. If you want to sit in your favorite easy chair and savor a novel or magazine, putting your shoes next to the chair can indicate to your family that you don't want to be disturbed. Be creative and, above all, respect your own boundaries and don't put them aside every time someone wants to chat.

YOUR PERSONAL NOTES ON PART TWO

Date: _____

_____

_____

_____

_____

_____

_____

_____

Date: _____

_____

_____

_____

_____

_____

_____

_____

Date: _____

_____

_____

_____

_____

_____

_____

_____

YOUR PERSONAL NOTES ON PART TWO

*Date:*_____

_____

_____

_____

_____

_____

_____

_____

*Date:*_____

_____

_____

_____

_____

_____

_____

_____

*Date:*_____

_____

_____

_____

_____

_____

_____

_____

Part Three: Inner World/Thoughts and Feelings

Part Three: Inner World/Thoughts and Feelings helps you explore how you think and feel about your world. It is important to assess these patterns because they influence your perceptions and govern your behaviors and decisions. They define your likes and dislikes, your judgments and opinions, and your general outlook on life. The six scales that relate to your Inner World act as filters that color and shape the way you classify and order experiences. Behaviors based on these perceptions have been learned and vary with individual expectations, environmental influences, life cycles, age, and personality traits.

Conflicts that arise from holding two contrary beliefs at the same time create inner tension and Inner World stress. For example, let's say that on the one hand you believe that a good mother should be at home full-time for her children, while on the other hand you know that, to provide the financial resources you need to care for your children properly, you must work outside the home. As a result, you feel torn apart, struggling to reconcile these two notions. Inner World conflicts must be resolved or mediated in order to reestablish an inner harmony.

Let's look at Mike Baxter again. Three of his four Burnouts lie in Part Three. That is no accident. His Scoring Grid shows a need to balance his Inner World with his real-life Environment. Scales 13, 14, and 15 reflect Inner World/Thoughts (beliefs, attitudes, rationalizations, and so on). Scales 16, 17, and 18 are Inner World/Feelings (emotions, gut-level reactions, values, for instance). It would be fair to say that Mike's view of the world is pessimistic, lacks a

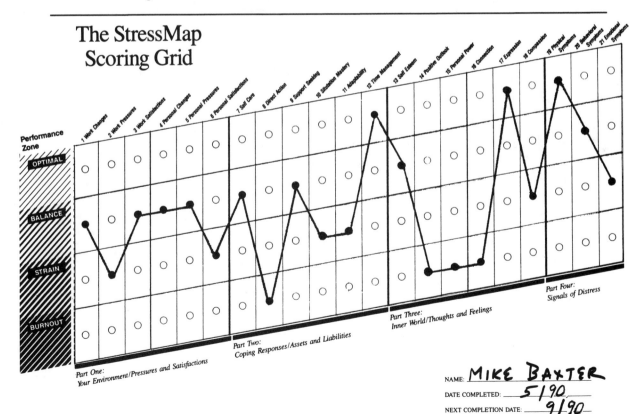

The StressMap Scoring Grid

NAME: MIKE BAXTER
DATE COMPLETED: 5/90
NEXT COMPLETION DATE: 9/90

sense of personal power, and has no strong central theme or feeling of connection. This world view may contribute to his inability to take Direct Action at this time.

Let's look at Maria Perez again. Her Part Three shows an even split between positive and negative patterns. Scales 13, 14, and 15 are all in Balance, all positive. These three scales measure the cognitive patterns that Maria uses to view the world. Despite heavy Personal Pressures and few Personal Satisfactions, she still feels relatively optimistic and maintains positive Self Esteem.

Her sense of Connection, Expression, and Compassion, however, indicates some Strain and is in need of attention. She may be attempting to be totally self sufficient and withdrawing and alienating herself from her inner circle of friends. This would explain her Burnout in Expression.

Now refer to your own Scoring Grid and ask yourself what conclusions you can draw about your own Inner World. Are your thinking patterns more positive than your feeling patterns? What other parts of your Scoring Grid do you think are most connected to this one?

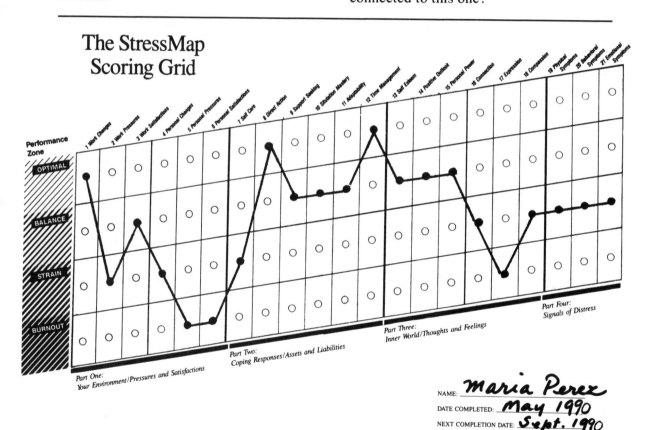

The StressMap Scoring Grid

NAME: *Maria Perez*
DATE COMPLETED: *May 1990*
NEXT COMPLETION DATE: *Sept. 1990*

SCALE **13**: Self Esteem

Definition

Self Esteem is an inner attitude of self respect, a sense of personal worth, and a state of valuing yourself. This attitude is reflected in a high, genuine, positive regard for yourself and for others. The opposite of Self Esteem is self criticism—a constant and ongoing cycle of self doubt, self blame, and dissatisfaction with your actions, abilities, and achievements.

Discussion

The Self Esteem scale measures how highly you value yourself. If you could stand outside yourself and observe how you spend your resources—time, money, and attention—what would you conclude? Do you value your friendships, your children, your car, your work? Are your spirit and productivity dampened by the unrealistic expectations, harsh demands, and negative opinions you place on yourself?

Self esteem is a sense of liking yourself, liking how you relate to others, feeling personally secure, and not having to prove your manhood or womanhood with external displays or symbols. Respecting others and having meaningful relationships affirm your right to have good things in your life. To bring love, excitement, and joy into your life, you must want these things and believe that you deserve them.

Our Self Esteem is influenced by many things—the environment we grew up in, the ways we were valued in our households, the role models we observed in our early life. Abused children and victims of domestic violence may find it difficult to correct very early attitudes toward their self worth. However, these negative self images must be turned into positive ones.

Poor Self Esteem is a factor in nearly every suicide. In fact, in her address to the American Orthopsychiatric Convention in 1987, psychologist Eliana Gill reported that low Self Esteem could be found at the root of many crimes of physical, sexual, and domestic abuse, as well as other kinds of destructive behavior. The state of California considers this issue so important that it has established a special Task Force on Self Esteem to address its relationship to crime reduction and social responsibility. The message is profoundly clear—loving yourself and knowing that you deserve and can create good things in your life are symbols of high Self Esteem. Compassion, which is strongly related to Self Esteem, will be discussed in Scale 18.

Tips for Improvement

● **Practice complimenting yourself often and genuinely.** Many of us have difficulty receiving praise or compliments from others. We feel embarrassed or undeserving. Practice accepting praise from others by praising yourself. Tell yourself, in a mirror if you wish, that you did a fine job on that dinner party, that you handled that difficult situation with your boss wonderfully. Be specific, and praise yourself in detail.

● **Do not allow others to diminish your personal self worth.** When interacting with superiors, customers, co-workers, or other associates, always remind yourself that you are OK, even when you make mistakes or could do better. If confronted with someone's anger or hostility, remember not to take this personally. Allow his or her comments to wash over you.

● **Do not use external factors to measure your self worth.** When our self worth is contingent on external factors—material goods, the status of our job, how much money we make, what others think about our accomplishments—we run the risk of feeling diminished or devastated if these factors change. Look inside yourself to the values you cherish and your inner source of personal power.

SCALE **14**: **Positive Outlook**

Definition

Positive Outlook is the ability to view the world with optimism and hope. This attitude shapes our expectations and experiences. The Optimal position reflects the ability to see the bright side of situations and to express beliefs for a favorable future consistently. The opposite of Positive Outlook is pessimism—the tendency to view the world as futile and gloomy and to expect the worst.

Discussion

You have a personal set of beliefs that has been shaped by past experiences and by what you have heard or been taught. This outlook influences your behavior in various situations. A pessimistic attitude, such as "Very little in life is fair," may lead to experiences that confirm this belief and hence set a vicious cycle in motion.

It is important to remember the power of language when talking to yourself or others. If you believe that you always get the short end of the stick, or that people rarely come through for you, you may set up the thoughts that mold your experiences. Your mind will take this message seriously and assume that, if this is what you think, then it is also what you want. For that reason it is important to direct your thoughts toward positive, rather than negative, expectations and outcomes. Since Positive Outlook is learned, you can actively choose to reshape your beliefs to be more positive and supportive of personal success.

Tips for Improvement

● **Take an honest inventory of your positive and negative attitudes.** Some of the beliefs we hold about ourselves and others empower us, while others limit or hinder us. Review your inventory and ask yourself where each of these outlooks came from. Were they learned from family, teachers, your own experiences, culture, environment, religion, or some other source? Understanding the origin of each outlook will help you put these attitudes in perspective, thus allowing you to evaluate, shift, or discard those that obstruct your positive performance.

● **Identify one outlook you wish to change.** Identify a recent situation in which your attitude got in the way of your success. Observe the language you use when you try to describe the situation today. Now try on a different attitude for the same situation. Imagine that you already act the way you wish you could. See it fully in great detail, and let yourself put it into action next time. This is called *mental rehearsal,* and it is a widely used form of preparation for athletic competition. Use mental rehearsal to eliminate self-defeating behaviors or habits that suppress optimism.

● **Replace negative with positive language.** Do you use a lot of absolutes—"always," "never," "right," and "wrong"? If this is the case, your outlook on life may be rigid and your responses to stressful situations may be routinely negative. Constant negative language reinforces negative expectations that minimize your chances for positive experiences. Try to see more possibilities than obstacles, and reward yourself for your skills, abilities, and achievements.

SCALE 15: Personal Power

Definition

Personal Power is knowing that you have the inner capacity to give and receive what you want and need. It is the ability to make things happen. Optimal performers have learned to tap this energy reservoir when they need it. It is enhanced by the belief or feeling that what you do makes a difference. The opposite of Personal Power is helplessness—feeling incapable to help yourself or fulfill your needs.

Discussion

Embracing Personal Power carries the responsibility of knowing how to use it. Many of the employee groups Essi Systems has worked with have felt negatively about power. When asked to brainstorm randomly about this topic, they respond with such words as: "force," "strength," "war," "oppression," "abuse," "masculine," "bullying," and "money." Rarely do they say "peace," "calm," "direction," or other words that connote more positive experiences of power. Personal Power involves finding the source of creativity and security that gives you the confidence to handle whatever comes up.

Personal Power allows you to take risks with a sense of excitement, and it fosters your potential for personal growth. It is knowing and accepting what you can and cannot control, and timing when and when not to act. Feeling in control is the best stress manager. People who suffer from Burnout or Strain on this scale tend to feel victimized and unable to cope.

Remember: using your own Personal Power does not detract from the Personal Power of others.

Tips for Improvement

● **Take action in situations you can control.** When you take action over things you can control, you have Situation Mastery (see Scale 10). When you take action in situations where you have no control you are practicing "ceaseless striving." When you do not take action on things over which you do have control, you are giving up, and when you don't have control and you don't take action you are letting go. Try to find situations over which you will have control, and take action. If you have no control, practice letting go.

● **Identify your patterns of powerlessness.** Become aware of those behaviors that contribute to powerlessness or helplessness in yourself. When do they arise? Are you at home? At work? Who is involved—your boss, colleagues, spouse, children? Ask yourself what part of this situation you can control and what action would most contribute to your well-being. Then take that action.

● **Question personal attitudes that limit your Personal Power.** A young girl and her mother were at the circus, and the child saw a huge elephant tied to a small wooden pole by a rather thin rope. She couldn't understand why the elephant didn't run off. The trainer explained that, when the elephant was very little, they used a wide steel post and big heavy chains to keep it from escaping. With every failed attempt to break free, the elephant grew more used to not trying, until now he never tries at all. Now the small chains are just as confining as the big ones were. The moral of the story: every once in a while, test the beliefs that once limited you. You might be surprised.

SCALE 16: Connection

Definition

Connection is a feeling of relatedness that links you to yourself, other people, and larger issues and questions. There is a purpose, fabric, or mission that weaves throughout your life and adds meaning to what you do. The opposite of Connection is alienation—feeling alone and detached from people and finding little meaning in life.

Discussion

Any task is less stressful when it is related to some important purpose. The desire to be the best parent or the most accomplished contributor to a given field may be the goal or mission that fuels your life. Whatever form the expression of this mission or higher purpose takes, the feeling is the same: "I am making a contribution, and what I am doing matters." Feeling that others value and appreciate your contribution also increases your performance.

Optimal performers on this scale are highly motivated, often feeling spiritually strengthened by their Connection, whether it be to a belief, cause, an ideology, a heritage, or a way of life. Connection brings tremendous Personal Satisfactions (Scale 6) and contributes to a strong Positive Outlook (Scale 14). Connection is the emotional counterpart of Positive Outlook.

Tips for Improvement

• **Record three of the strongest needs in your life right now.** Ask yourself how they are being met. Examine the core values or beliefs around which these needs revolve, and find ways of fulfilling them.

• **Put your body, time, and money where your beliefs are.** Connection is value-based, and it requires more than espousing a point of view over cocktails. Throw yourself passionately into something you value or hold dear, show up at a meeting, donate to a cause you believe in, volunteer to help. *Act on what you say is important.*

• **Do something daily to reinforce your Connection to your central purpose or mission.** Take time every day, if only for a moment, to remind yourself of what's important to you, and take some action that expresses it. Let one motorist cut in front of you without yelling at him or her, for example. See that gesture as a step toward world peace. Take a daily inventory of one thing you did today toward meeting a life goal or one of the needs you listed above. Tell someone you are glad he or she is in your life.

• **Bring more self expression into your work and play.** Risk being unique, and display your many talents and abilities. If you are passionate about a cause, an idea, a song, let people know. Strengthen relationships with the people closest to you. Imagine you have been told you have six months to live. What would you do? What would you say to others? Whom would you say it to? Don't wait.

• **Take an active role in finding a group whose work and/or activities you enjoy.** As we grew up, our lives were centered on groups that we were born into—our families, neighborhoods, local schools, religious groups, etc. Over the years, however, we may have moved away or our beliefs and values may have changed. When this happens, we need to take responsibility for finding new communities to live within. If you feel a need for a spiritual community, attend services or meetings and notice when one feels right. Whatever your interest, there are others who share it. Do research, look in the phone book, ask friends. Sharing enjoyed activities and values provides us with a valuable sense of connection to others and the world.

SCALE **17**: **Expression**

Definition

Expression is sharing what you think and feel through direct and indirect communication with others. The opposite of Expression is internalization which is when you keep thoughts and feelings inside, sometimes hiding them even from yourself.

Discussion

Expression poses some risk for people who have had little experience with being vulnerable or sharing deeply held beliefs with others. Many of us fear ridicule or rejection if we reveal our desires, needs, or wants to others. But not letting people know if and when you disagree with them, and withdrawing and avoiding others when you are upset, are coping strategies that may be counterproductive. Self disclosure is really the only way for those closest to you to know exactly what you want, or how you wish to receive it; you must express that information at least once. Partners in a relationship very often expect each other to know what they want or need, often using indecipherable messages that are intended to inform, yet serve only to confuse. Too often, the end result of this is frustrated expectations and a sense of not being able to get what they want.

In the many groups Essi Systems has interviewed, this scale shows very distinct male-female differences. The cultural stereotypes of strength and silence as desirable masculine traits, and intuition, expression, and emotionalism as undesirable feminine traits, inhibit both men and women from expressing themselves fully.

Tips for Improvement

• **Find multiple avenues for self expression.** Whether verbal or nonverbal, direct or indirect, it is important to find some channel for communicating your thoughts and feelings. Keeping a journal, drawing, dancing, playing an instrument, composing a tune, writing a poem, cooking, participating in sports—all of these are healthy forms of self expression.

• **Discover your personal style of expression.** No two people are exactly alike. Find your personal style or trademark, such as developing a collection of frogs, always sending flowers to cheer up others during hard times, or wearing colorful clothes.

SCALE **18**: **Compassion**

Definition

Compassion is the capacity to empathize with other people, seeing their point of view and recognizing their strengths and limits. The opposite of Compassion is resentment—holding on to anger about yourself, another person, or your circumstances to the point of bitterness or hostility.

Discussion

To resent is to show displeasure and indignation at some act or remark that is perceived as injurious or offensive. Excessive anger or hostility can cause emotional paralysis and may contribute to such health problems as heart disease, high blood pressure, and other cardiovascular dysfunctions.

Compassion, on the other hand, allows you to feel for another person's situation or plight. It requires learning to forgive yourself and others for not being perfect. Compassionate behaviors are symbols of high self esteem and the ability to let go of unreasonable jealousies and judgments.

Scoring in the Optimal zone on this scale shows a high level of commiseration and acceptance of individual differences. Burnout is marked by the desire to punish as an attempt to right some sense of being wronged. Blaming others, being impatient, being cruel, ridiculing others, and losing your temper regularly are characteristics of poor performance on this scale.

Anger is sometimes mixed with an undercurrent of other feelings, such as sadness, hurt, or fear. Failure to identify these secondary feelings intensifies the expression of anger and makes it difficult to communicate this emotion in a way that lets others respond with Compassion.

Tips for Improvement

● **Look beyond surface anger or resentment and discover the feelings underneath.** To say, "I'm angry," may be one way of labeling what may be a less obvious, but nonetheless intense, feeling of sadness, hurt, rejection, betrayal, or fear. Be more willing to learn and use words that describe these underlying feelings, and avoid the temptation to ignore or deny them. Take a moment when you feel upset or bitter to ask yourself what you are feeling. Try expressing this feeling, instead of anger, to another person.

● **Learn to forgive yourself for not being perfect.** Very often the things we ridicule in others are precisely those things we dislike in ourselves. Identify frustration and bitterness directed toward yourself. Make allowances for your limitations and other people's, and let go of critical, demeaning, and punitive self talk. Remind yourself that mistakes are part of learning, and are not reflections of your self worth. (See Scale 13, Self Esteem.)

● **Evaluate behaviors, not people, when stating your dislikes.** When expressing disagreement with others, whether it be over politics, religion, or ways to approach a work or family problem, focus on the issues being discussed, not the person discussing it. Say, "I disagree with your opinion," not, "I think you are stupid to think that way." When expressing your feelings, take responsibility for these emotions and allow others to do the same. Use "I" statements that embrace this responsibility, not "you" statements, which put you in the power of others. For example, say, "I feel hurt," instead of, "You hurt me."

YOUR PERSONAL NOTES ON PART THREE

Date: _____

_____

_____

_____

_____

_____

_____

_____

Date: _____

_____

_____

_____

_____

_____

_____

_____

Date: _____

_____

_____

_____

_____

_____

_____

YOUR PERSONAL NOTES ON PART THREE

Date: _____

_____

_____

_____

_____

_____

_____

_____

Date: _____

_____

_____

_____

_____

_____

_____

_____

Date: _____

_____

_____

_____

_____

_____

_____

_____

Part Four: Signals of Distress

Part Four: Signals of Distress reflects the traditional measures of poor stress management and ineffective coping responses. There are three distinct ways you can experience chronic stress build-up: physically, behaviorally, and emotionally. Most of us show some tendency to manifest stress in one way more than in the others, but you can show signs of distress in all three categories simultaneously.

For many people, the first awareness of stress come through body signals, in the form of illnesses, colds, allergy attacks, aches, pains, and muscle cramps or strains. When any of these comes to your attention, you may be showing signs of Strain or Burnout in your stress-management efforts. The *StressMap* Questionnaire can help you identify others areas of coping that should be bolstered to lessen your distress.

Stress can also manifest itself behavior-ally, as we act out ways of relieving or denying stress. People who demonstrate this tendency may report a different set of reactions to stress: erratic eating, drug abuse, withdrawing from support, and excessive drinking. Accidents and injuries are sure signs of inadequate coping or concern during stressful times.

Finally, stress can manifest itself emotionally, through the body's nervous system. Crying easily, fidgeting, insomnia, inability to concentrate, angry outbursts, and loss of sexual interest are all symptoms of emotional distress.

It is important to listen carefully to your own physical, behavioral, and emotional symptoms and not wait until they cause bodily damage or serious health problems. (Note: any symptom on these three scales that you observe every day may require professional or medical attention.)

Using the same Scoring Grid when you retake StressMap in another three or four months can show you areas of improvement or new problems.

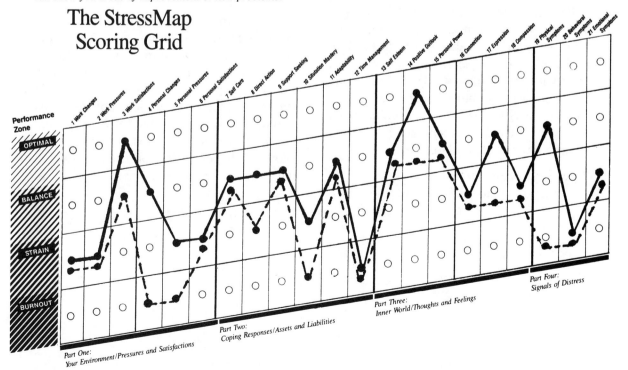

The StressMap Scoring Grid

SCALE 19: Physical Symptoms

Definition

Physical Symptoms are the bodily manifestations of chronic or excessive stress in the form of pain, disorder, or illness. In the Optimal position, this scale represents good health and physical well-being; in the Burnout position, breakdown and severe disrepair.

Discussion

Think of Physical Symptoms as the things your body does in response to the stress in your life. The untuned body, or the body lacking in healthy Self Care practices, cannot withstand day-to-day wear and tear and will show signs of distress. Back pain, muscle tension, skin rashes, colds, allergy flare-ups, diarrhea, constipation, and sore throats may all be related to some unaddressed perception of stress.

Repeated experiences of stress without release or relaxation develop into Physical Symptoms of distress that may aggravate or cause complex health problems. The minor symptoms mentioned above cost millions of dollars in unnecessary visits to hospitals and physicians' offices every year. Too often we seek medical solutions to lifestyle problems, without learning new ways to cope with stress in day-to-day living. While any chronic symptom may stem from causes other than stress, research suggests that more than 70 percent of all physical symptoms are stress-related.

Tips for Improvement

● **Identify the particular way in which your body shows stress.** Perhaps your stress manifests itself with muscular problems—cramping, tightening in the shoulders, or back pain. Perhaps you show your stress through the digestive or excretory system with diarrhea, constipation, or acid stomach. Being attentive to the particular ways your body exhibits stress can help you identify stressful situations before they do you too much harm.

● **Develop effective ways of telling your body that you are *not* being attacked.** The body has no way of knowing the difference between real and imagined danger. If you are constantly mobilizing your body's defenses to release hormones and chemicals to protect you in the event of attack, but never let your guard down when the threat has passed, then your stress level, or readiness, stays on red alert and keeps your body at emergency pitch. A constant state of red alert with no sign of release causes physical deterioration and ultimately leads to physical breakdown.

● **Become fully absorbed in some activity other than the one you do every day.** If you are a stockbroker used to the stress of quick decisions and fast turnarounds, then go on a rafting trip on the rapids, or engage in some other activity that does not allow you to think about anything but the task at hand, like maneuvering the next turn or staying afloat. Shift your attention from survival in the corporate mode to survival in a physical mode.

SCALE **20**: **Behavioral Symptoms**

Definition

Behavioral Symptoms are the regular, usually self-defeating, ways in which we act to relieve or escape tension and pressure. The behaviors we choose will greatly contribute to our state of health. In the Optimal position, the choices we make contribute to our resilience; in the Burnout position, they contribute to dependency and addiction.

Discussion

Smoking, excessive or unwise use of medication and other drugs, overeating, eating poorly, watching more than two hours of television a day, and distractedness to the degree that it causes injuries or accidents are all examples of unhealthy behavioral reactions to daily stress. When seriously indulged, they can actually *increase* stress and cause additional health and interpersonal problems. It is much easier to space out in front of the television than it is to talk to your spouse about a problem in your relationship. Withdrawing from close relationships, resenting people you encounter at work, feeling overwhelmed by work or home commitments, and having difficulty completing tasks may all signal a need to find other ways of dealing with your stress. Furthermore, these behaviors do nothing to change or manage the source of the tension.

In the Strain and Burnout positions, people typically report feeling unable to handle stress and bury their helplessness in destructive behaviors. They become psychologically (as well as physically) addicted to these tension releasers, which include drug dependence, bruxism (gnashing of teeth), lethargy, and eating disorders.

Tips for Improvement

● **Identify self-defeating behaviors.** Look at your own self-defeating behavior patterns. Ask yourself how you feel when you resort to one. Is this action an attempt to cope with tension or stress in some way? Does it help you relieve, forget, avoid, or escape something else? First learn what the desired state is and see if you can begin to achieve that state through other, less destructive activities.

● **Formulate a realistic plan for making change.** Choose the one practice you are most willing to consider changing. It doesn't have to be your "worst" symptom, but you do have to choose one that you actively desire to modify or alter, such as watching too much television. Use the Action-Planning Worksheet (page 73) to develop a realistic plan for change.

● **Use a buddy system to change behaviors.** Seek support from your family and friends to change these behaviors. Select someone as a helper or confidant to check in with. Using a buddy system can help both of you get through difficult periods of adjustment.

● **Seek professional assistance for dependency treatment.** You may wish to seek professional assistance if you find that you are fully dependent on some substance or behavior, such as alcohol, other drugs, or food. Find out whether your workplace has an Employee Assistance Program, and take advantage of the resources it offers.

SCALE 21: **Emotional Symptoms**

Definition

Emotional Symptoms are subjective re-actions to stress and pressure that, if left unchecked, can result in disorders of the central nervous system. These symptoms linger, impair performance, and they drain both physical and psychological energy re-serves.

Discussion

Everyone experiences strong emotion when under pressure. Most people find av-enues for its expression, though, which allow the body to rebound and respond to the situation. When that expression or re-lease of emotion is not adequate to the amount of stress, residual pressure remains. Doubts, fears, and worries about inadequa-cies can linger and be reinforced through negative self talk. Rehashing a mistake or failure in your mind triggers an emotional reaction, which the body in turn interprets as a threat of harm or danger.

The body will respond chemically and emotionally, whether the danger is real or imagined. The result may be tremors, tics, apathy, fatigue, or exhaustion. Depression, fearfulness, irritability, angry outbursts, anxiety, or feeling keyed up are all signals that some of your emotional coping mechan-isms may not be working well. Over time you develop patterns of overreacting or un-derreacting to stressful situations. These create chronic emotional upset. These ex-treme emotions are usually accompanied by self criticism and helplessness. People in the Burnout or Strain zones may also turn to substance abuse (tranquilizers or alcohol) to alleviate their distress.

Tips for Improvement

● **Connect emotional symptoms to their sources.** Review your list of Emotional Symptoms, and note any items that you ex-perience nearly every day or every week. Identify as best you can the situations that trigger these symptoms. Are they issues at work? Home? An upcoming deadline? An inconsiderate roommate? What could you do to change that situation practically? By looking beyond the immediate surface symptom, you can gain insights into what you will need to reduce the stress. Learn how to deep-breathe, do yoga, meditate, ex-ercise regularly, get a massage, stop nega-tive self talk, seek help from your support systems—do whatever it takes to help you get rid of these symptoms and bolster your emotional and psychic energy.

● **Learn to let go of events beyond your control.** Many people subject themselves to impossible deadlines, unachievable goals, and unreasonable time schedules. This type of regimen sabotages their chances for suc-cess and creates chaos for both these people and those around them. Keep perspective on pressures by knowing where and when not to take action. Control those factors you can do something about, and set realistic timetables for achieving your goals. Respect your emotional needs for safety, play, and relaxation, and give yourself a daily dose of these tension reducers. As the slogan goes, "You deserve a break today." Give your-self one.

YOUR PERSONAL NOTES ON PART FOUR

Date: _____

_____

_____

_____

_____

_____

_____

_____

Date: _____

_____

_____

_____

_____

_____

_____

_____

Date: _____

_____

_____

_____

_____

_____

_____

_____

YOUR PERSONAL NOTES ON PART FOUR

Date: _____

_____

_____

_____

_____

_____

_____

_____

Date: _____

_____

_____

_____

_____

_____

_____

_____

Date: _____

_____

_____

_____

_____

_____

_____

_____

Action-Planning Worksheet

1. Describe the behavior or situation you wish to change.

_____

_____

_____

_____

_____

2. How do you presently respond? (What do you think, feel, and do in that situation?)

_____

_____

_____

_____

3. How would you like to respond? (What would change about how you think, feel, or act in that situation? What is your goal?)

_____

_____

_____

_____

4. List as many ideas and actions as you can for meeting your goals. (Identify alternative solutions, brainstorm.)

_____

_____

_____

_____

(Now go back and circle the alternative that you think is the best way for you to reach your goal.)

(CONTINUED OVERLEAF)

5. What might hinder you from reaching your goals? (negative self talk, time constraints, etc.?)

_____

_____

_____

6. What might help you in reaching your goals? (people, resources, new skills, etc.?)

_____

_____

_____

7. What specific steps are you willing to take to create change? By when? (date?)

_____

_____

_____

8. Whom will you ask to help or support you in achieving your goal?

_____

_____

_____

_____

9. How will you reward yourself when you have accomplished your goals?

_____

_____

_____

I commit myself to accomplish (specific change)

_____

_____

_____

Signature   _Date_

The Workplace Challenge

More and more corporations are faced with difficult questions and concerns regarding how to get work done through others. Employee confidentiality, rights to privacy, invasive inquiries into personal habits and home life, individual lifestyle choices that affect health and medical insurance that our companies pay for—where do we draw the lines? The company as teacher, trainer, and coach—roles that employees welcome and might even expect—has drawn criticism and alarm when employees sense the company prying, intruding, or controlling their personal freedoms.

The workplace challenge for corporations is to motivate employees and produce goods and services while maintaining the role of manager, respecting the individual, and valuing the diversities of new American workers. The challenge is to find innovative ways to teach self-empowerment and to enable employees to achieve levels of optimal performance and job satisfaction.

These concerns have most definitely been debated in the health and wellness arenas. Company health-care plans, long and short term disability plans, and worker compensation costs have risen dramatically in the last 10 years. Out of control increases in medical care have caused the American corporation to ponder questions of how to improve both profitability and employee performance.

The implications are very important. On the one hand, American organizations are locked in a difficult struggle for economic survival in the marketplace jungle outside their walls; on the other hand, companies are straining to keep employees healthy, productive, and loyal inside their walls. The solutions are complicated, yet one avenue that has gained support in the last few years has been the concept of self-care. When employees are given the tools they need to take care of themselves, they do. Finding high quality self-measuring and reporting devices is an essential first step towards installing self-management concepts. The most versatile tools can allow employees anonymity while providing the organization with valuable composite information for making improvements.

Putting StressMap *to Use in Companies*

Many of the more than 1500 corporations and organizations in the United States who have used *StressMap* have emphasized its confidential nature and ease of implementation. Even when incorporated into existing stress management programs as a strict assessment device, human resource professionals report they can still accomplish their important learning objectives without asking employees to divulge personal scoring information

Physicians, nurses, therapists, counselors, chiropractors, and health and fitness professionals use *StressMap* on a one-on-one basis to analyze stress/performance strengths and weaknesses in conjunction with the usual health risk appraisals like cardiovascular testing and overall body fitness measurements. One large clothing manufacturer incorporates the *Map* in its intake process for its fitness center. When goal-setting sessions for individual fitness plans are conducted with the exercise physiologist, nutritionist, and registered nurse, *StressMap* becomes integral to identifying problems and planning holistic improvements in lifestyle. Learning new, more reasonable time management skills or rebalancing work and home priorities, items easily identified through using *StressMap,* can make the difference in maintaining physical health.

A chiropractor in Boston administers *StressMap* to patients who are caught in a cycle of treatment and relapse beyond which they have difficulty advancing. *StressMap* gives this practitioner and her patients the information they both need to understand the details of this particular pattern and to develop a treatment plan the patients can stick to. When we take our bodies literally we might ask: What is my back saying to me? What can't I stand? What back-up do I need? This chiropractor reports great success with this approach, because patients feel listened to and the whole person is considered in the treatment plan.

An Atlanta-based telecommunications company approached Essi Systems with the request to design and recommend a usable stress management program for 200 of its people. They had determined that stress was a serious problem, since work stress was on the lips of most employees. Like many organizations we work with, this one had conducted an employee survey asking a myriad of questions regarding the work environment and the perceptions of the workforce. *StressMap* asks 28 questions concerning job pressures, 9 questions on work changes, and 15 questions on work satisfactions. That's 52 questions, each different, to attempt to pinpoint the nature and sources of work stress. Because of this, we were able to target the core of employee problem areas, and design solutions that went to the heart of the matter. Instead of offering an 8-hour program to teach higher level skills like deep muscle relaxation and visualization, which require long-term practice and commitment, this company started with a *StressMap* campaign to help employees identify their most pressing sources of distress in the tool's 4 major parts. Given the limited internal resources of this organization, we recommended the creation of a referral directory to community services and low or sliding scale fee services in the area.

In addition, 90 minute interpretation sessions, on company time, were offered to employees to better understand the functions and intricacies of the *StressMap* grid, detailing the information most relevant to each individual's health level and patterns of distress. Further, a two day *StressMap* Certification Workshop with the Personnel Director and staff enabled employes to implement and present the program themselves, ultimately getting *StressMap* into the hands of all 200 employees.

This workshop attained a full 46 percent utilization rate. Participants reported feeling satisfied and left the session with clear plans for making improvements that were well-defined and achievable. In 3 months they could prepare to retest and see the fruits of their efforts.

The self-care approach espouses self-management and self-responsibility for personal health and optimal work performance. The employers we work with are willing to share the obligation for keeping the work environment and operating structures responsive to the ever-changing needs of their employees and the demands of the contemporary marketplace.

Coping With A Changing World

We're living in a time of great and rapid social, economic, and cultural change—and change, although inevitable, necessitates varying degrees of adjustment.

Take a look around you. Daily newspapers tell us about the shift from a national to a global economy; social changes make headlines everywhere. And if you're reading this book, chances are you're feeling the effects of distress in your own life. The fact is, change is hard. We tend to like the familiar, whether it's good for us or not, because it's safe and comfortable. It's like an old glove—it seems to fit, or it once did—and our experience of its comfort is enhanced by the memories that surround it.

In today's world, however, much of what was once familiar is changing as a result of economic, social, and cultural forces that are beyond our immediate control. We consequently find ourselves in the midst of great unrest, working to adjust successfully to a number of potentially distressful situations.

Let's take a look at the stressors that are affecting us at work and at home.

Many people have been directly affected by the restructuring and downsizing implemented by their employers in this age of mergers and acquisitions. In this climate, a corporation tends to adjust its internal system to accommodate an external economy in flux. Often the resulting "mean and lean" stance negates a lifetime alliance between employee and employer and doesn't take into consideration the human cost incurred. Change managers seem unconscious of the shift in values they have brought about in employees who have lost jobs, seniority, or stability through reorganization. In such an atmosphere, employees of all levels have begun to place loyalty to self above loyalty to company. They have made a shift in life priorities. They have clarified, for themselves, a set of personal values based on life experience.

A desire for greater job satisfaction is one way this trend toward loyalty to self over loyalty to one's employer shows up in the workforce. Increasingly, money is seen as inadequate compensation for meaningless work. People affected by this loyalty shift also tend to give their families and friends a more prominent place in their lives than they did before making this kind of value-based change.

In many families, financial pressures have made it necessary for both parents to work. Most women must be employed outside the home to support themselves and their families, bringing millions into the workforce, in itself a major social change. Women are also discovering in work a new sense of self and an expanded definition of power. They find they can run companies, be vice presidents of marketing, lobbyists, scientists, or executives.

The very nature of the term "family" has changed. Today we have "blended" families due to remarriages and adoption, single parent families, nuclear families, and non-traditional families. The role of parenthood has changed, as have the roles of men and women in relationships. There's also more parity between adult members of families of all types. The issue of childcare for two-career families and single parents adds additional distress.

Life roles that were once clearly defined have become increasingly ambiguous for everyone, regardless of age, race, gender, or culture. The boundary that used to separate our work and home identities has been made permeable by the influx of women into the workplace and the changes in family structure.

In the face of all this change—and potential distress—what do we do? We've never been taught to deal with so many rapid changes. How do we cope? In an environment where social, economic, and cultural structures are in flux, the challenge is to make choices that maintain one's integrity. To be stable today and experience stress in a positive way, we need to know what we believe and what our values are—for the changing nature of the world around us is less likely to offer us the anchor of tradition that many of us have looked to for security in years past. We need to find security within ourselves. How do we do this? By learning who we are, what we value, what we love to do, and what kind of life we really want. Sonia Johnson, author of *Going Out of Our Minds,* would suggest that we need to learn to shift the question from "What am I going to *do?*" to "How am I going to *be?*" In other words, how will I conduct myself, how will I live my life?

To live in today's world in good health we need to *be* stress hardy. One study examined 200 business executives at Illinois Bell Telephone Company who had undergone great distress during the AT&T divestiture. University of Chicago psychologists Suzanne Kobasa and Salvatore Maddi identified the "three C's" necessary for stress hardiness as manifested by the 100 executives who reported few signs of illness.

They had a sense of *control* over their work lives and felt that through their attitudes "they could control the impact of the problems [at work] if not the problems themselves."

They possessed a sense of *commitment* to and valued their work and personal relationships, which gave them a sense of "meaning, direction and excitement."

They saw change as a *challenge* and an "opportunity for growth and learning."

At Essi Systems we've added another "C" to the "three C's" of Kobasa and Maddi—personal *centeredness*—for we believe that this characteristic is essential for successful coping with today's stressors. When you're centered, you know yourself and feel connected to your personal power. You know what your values are and you use them as "anchors" to create a strong base from which to live your life, even when choices are difficult. Being centered means that deep within you know you have the capacity to both take care of yourself and to manage what life brings. You're integrated: your body, mind, emotions, and spiritual self all work as one to provide you with answers to life's questions. When you're centered, you listen to your internal voice and are able to hear when it says, "Ah ha! That's the way I need to go"— even when it's hard.

Knowing what your values are and feeling secure in your ability to enjoy the complexity of life in the modern jungle are both essential skills for effective stress management. These skills are like tools: you can reach into your toolbox and pull out the coping skill that best matches a particular life situation. When you live from a place of personal centeredness, you value who you are, for knowing what you're about requires a lot of self-examination and questioning of past beliefs and values. Each day you have to be willing to ask, "Is this what I want? Is this me? Or is this something that my mother [or partner, father, or someone else] wants or wanted for me?"

Knowing who you are means knowing what you want, being willing and able to take care of yourself, and asking for what you want and need. It requires a lot of work, but the rewards are great.

You know what's good for *you*. You're not at the mercy of ever-present outside influences such as other people's expectations, events at work, or constant bombardment by media models. At your center, you value yourself as a person regardless of externals. This is personal centeredness.

Successfully dealing with stress also means remaining adaptable. It is, of course, normal to feel fear and anxiety when facing change and the unknown. It's healthy. We all feel this way. But being adaptable and flexible is a skill you can learn that will help you see change as an opportunity for growth and learning.

Personal centeredness, commitment, challenge, and control are part of your stress tool kit that you can use in any situation. We use these "4 C's" to cope with three kinds of stress-producing change.

The simplest are changes in routine and ritual. For example, if your dry cleaner moves 15 blocks to a new location, your Saturday errand-running will need modification. You might even automatically drive to the cleaner's old store a few times before you get used to going to her new address. Changes in routine and ritual are identifiable, contained in a single issue, and are measurable (e.g., either you use the same cleaner or you don't). This kind of change is often a hassle, but seen in the big picture is relatively easy to cope with.

Another kind of change is event-initiated. Some event-initiated changes require major adjustments in our lives, while others take smaller adjustments. Questions about this type of change appear in this book on *StressMap* scale four and measure the amount of distress a person is experiencing in her or his life. A new job, divorce, marriage, a change of residence, or the death of a relative or even a pet all fall into this category. These events are associated with a "marker"—the day of the accident, the weekend you got married, or the winter you bought your home.

However, the event by itself is not an adequate measure of the distress it might cause. The event must be considered in relation to you. The amount of time needed for adjustment, the intensity of the feeling experienced, and the ability to manage the transition that the event requires is totally dependent on you, your natural cycle, and the choices you make. A similar event can be experienced by two people in very different ways, depending on their perspectives. For example, one woman might see her divorce as a liberating event, while for another it may be devastating. The effect of an event-initiated change in a person's life depends both on the event itself *and* its relationship to the person affected.

The third type of change we experience is a value-based change. When you make a value-based change, you're trying to bring your actions into alignment with what you value. Value-based changes are personal changes, because they reflect a shift in what we feel is important. They can begin as a result of an external event or an internal shift. Value-based changes occur because we choose to make them.

We are not born with a set of values that remain constant throughout our lives. As children, most of us adopt the value system that our parents give us. In some families, the value of education is emphasized. In others, a prevailing value might be "always exercise your voting rights."

When we take the values of our parents for our own, we keep them until they no longer serve us. Young adults, in their quest for separation and independence, frequently reject many of the values they have learned at home. Later, after varying amounts of life experience, they sometimes readopt some of these values, modifying them to fit their own view of life.

The values of a child are clearly different from those of a

teenager; and the values of a teenager, who might feel nothing is more important than her peer group's Saturday night bash, change as she matures and becomes more interested in the company of one person than in the companionship of her crowd. As we grow, we change and constantly reexamine our values, asking ourselves "What's important to me now?" and "How do I want to live my life?"

Your Values

Since values are intangible, we've come up with three clues that will clarify what we mean. These clues will also assist you in clarifying your own values and will help you identify the values of others as well.

Remember that people act on whatever is important to them. If you're a supervisor, a parent, a teacher, or anyone who deals with people in general, you need to be able to listen and watch for these clues because values motivate behavior. We use the word "clues" rather than a word like "rules" because it's impossible to make a definitive statement or judgment as to what value is being spoken to by a person's language, symbols, or action. We can get only a glimmer of the value, since people will often surprise you— and sometimes themselves as well!

Clue #1: Our values are always identified by our language. Notice when you say, "I love this," "I cherish that," "This is important to me," "I detest that," or "I must have this." These verbal clues name what we feel is or is not important.

For example, someone might say, "I love this old house." We know that there's something important being said about this old house, but we don't know exactly what the value is. Perhaps the memories associated with the house are significant, or maybe the speaker grew up in the house or built it. We don't know the specific source of the value, or precisely what it is. But we *do* know that there's something of importance being spoken to here.

Clue #2: The symbols we use and surround ourselves with also identify values. The ring someone wears could be a symbol of commitment, the car someone drives a symbol of social status. Your hairstyle can also speak to personal value.

Clue #3: How we behave or act is another value identifier. What we strive for and what we avoid also show what we value.

For example, if you were to see a father decline an invitation to go sailing with his buddies because he's going to take his daughters to the zoo, you wouldn't have to hear him say, "My daughters are important to me," to understand from his actions that his daughters *are* important to him.

In another example, we see a woman in an office who always

remembers everyone's birthday. She organizes each celebration, buying the cake, making sure everyone signs the card, etc. With these actions, she shows that something here is important to her. It might be the value of remembering birthdays, or of helping friends feel valued, or of wanting to feel valued herself when her own birthday comes up.

Sometimes people show what they value through their avocations. A pilot may like the thrill of adventure in the air, or the rush she gets flying into the clouds. Although you might not necessarily know *what* it is that the pilot likes about her sport, you could know that every Saturday morning she gets up and takes lessons to learn how to fly. The way a person spends his or her time, in this case, flying, is another way to find out what someone values.

It's wise to remember that when you make a value-based change, it will touch all spheres of your life. Sometimes this kind of change is precipitated by an event. For example, a 15-year manager for a large organization loses his job in a messy corporate merger. When he finds another job he regains his self-esteem but no longer feels a sense of great loyalty to any employer. He has shifted his allegiance from his employer to himself. As a result of this shift, he begins to question the things he feels are important in life and no longer sees his self-esteem defined by the strength or failure of the corporation that he works for. One such manager described his shift in this way:

"I always thought that hard work and perseverance would protect me from layoffs. When the company let me go I was devastated. I felt lost and worthless. I made up my mind right then that I would bring more fun and enjoyment into my life and would no longer rely solely on my job for my self-esteem or feelings of personal worth. Since I've made this shift, if I'm asked whether I want to work overtime or go to the ballgame, there's no question which I'd choose. The ballgame, of course!"

He now places more value on his personal life and his family and friends. They, he feels, are what really matter. This man has made a value-based change.

The decision of a problem drinker to stop drinking is also a value-based change. An active drinker will do whatever is necessary to make sure alcohol is a part of his or her life. This is a priority. However, when this person decides to become clean and sober, his or her values shift. The value of being alcohol-free overrides everything. Living each day without alcohol affects every part of the nondrinker's life: how one deals with conflict without alcohol, who one associates with, who one befriends. Abstinence replaces out-of-control drinking. This person must find new ways of dealing with emotions and bring his or her behavior into alignment with a new value system.

Value-based change produces a special group of stressors in

our lives. We're bombarded by "shoulds"—we "should" be doing better, we "should" be making more progress. Be patient and gentle with yourself while making this type of change, for its effects are profound and will, for a while, be a source of overwhelming new feelings in your life.

Those around you will also react to the new you. Many will react negatively and feel threatened by your desire for change and your ability to work towards creating the life you want for yourself. Others will be encouraging, viewing your development as a positive step. Include them in the supportive environment you create for yourself. Learn to go slow and make sure that work and play both contribute to your sense of personal centeredness.

As we all know, change is difficult. Whether it's the result of external circumstances or the result of an internal, value-based change, it's bound to produce discomfort and challenge in our lives. We can protect ourselves from many of the health-threatening effects of distress by developing the characteristics of stress hardiness: commitment, challenge, control, and, most important, personal centeredness.

A WORD
ABOUT THE RESEARCH

Product testing and research into the norms, reliability, and validity of the *StressMap* scales were conducted with nearly 400 employees throughout 1984 and 1985.

RELIABILITY

In designing a viable assessment tool, the first question is whether the scales are statistically reliable; that is, do the questions consistently measure the factors being explored. Dr. Karen Trocki's findings were very clear: all 21 *StressMap* scales have reliability coefficients that are more than adequate, with a range from .72 to .93. As a general rule, the more items in a scale, the easier it is to attain a high reliability coefficient. The challenge was to create concise scales while maintaining high reliability. This achievement was confirmed when the reliability coefficients fell into the high .70's on the Inner World scales, which have only 8 to 11 items each.

NORMS

The second goal of our research was to establish a preliminary set of norms, the standard average or median achievement based on the respondent group. These figures would determine the numerical weighting for each of the four Performance Zones. Unlike other measurement tools, *StressMap* norms would represent a wide variety of employed people with no particular stress-related problems or illnesses. This would ensure that the *StressMap* norms reflect the performance levels of a relatively varied and healthy group of working men and women.

VALIDITY

The third research question, and perhaps the most important, is whether *StressMap* is valid. Do the scales of *StressMap* actually measure behavior that relates to people's ability to manage stress? All of the original research was taken from studies whose measures and statistical findings had been strictly scrutinized, tested, and proven. We further determined validity through a comparison of *StressMap's* last three scales, Part Four: Signals of Distress (the outcomes of poor stress management and a traditional measure of difficulty in coping with stress) to the scores on each of the other 18 scales. Again our findings showed that each of the first 18 scales was linked to degree of healthiness in the Signals of Distress and was therefore a valid instrument.

StressMap also has an extremely high degree of "face validity," which means that the factor being measured can be easily identified by any person taking it. Most respondents were concerned that the questions "fit" their real-life stress experiences at home and at work.

COMPARISON OF DEMOGRAPHICS AND SCALE SCORES

Here are several interesting points of information from a comparison of demographics and scale scores:

- Older respondents reported fewer symptoms (Scales 19–21) and pressures (Scales 2 and 5). Perhaps some of this can be explained by the correlation of age and experience. Learning to take things as they come or realizing one will survive can be a stress reliever.

- Women reported more changes (Scales 1 and 4), more family pressures, and more stress symptoms than men. They scored lower on Adaptability (Scale 11) and Time

Management (Scale 12). It can be speculated that women are more willing to express their feelings, are more self critical, and are expected to fill more roles.

- Different occupations and companies clearly had different stress levels. Teachers noted the highest stress symptoms and Work Pressures, as well as low work support. A company in considerable transition had the next highest level of overall stress.

RESEARCH BACKGROUND

Part One

The first area of measurement, Your Environment/Pressures and Satisfactions, includes both work and family environments. For both work and family there are separate scales for change, pressures, and satisfactions. The first four scales on work and Personal Changes draw from Holmes and Rahe's life-change research. Scales 2, Work Pressures, and 5, Personal Pressures, draw from several work-pressure and environmental scales, using work-stress research by MacLean, job-role and strain research by Katz and Kahn, and other common work-environment scales. The satisfaction scales, especially family satisfaction scales, draw from Moos' research on family support. The pressure and satisfaction scales also draw from Lazarus's hassle and uplift research.

Part Two

The second area deals with coping resources and responses and includes six scales. These are Self Care, Direct Action, Support Seeking, Situation Mastery, Flexibility, and Time Management. Scale 7, Self Care, stems from health-habits research, especially the studies of Belloc, Breslow, Syme, and Berkman. The coping skills draw on research on coping styles by Lazarus. Scale 8, Direct Action, comes from Wallston's locus-of-control studies. Scale 9, Support Seeking, comes from social-support research by Cobb, Berkman, and others, and Scale 10, Situation Mastery, draws on the many Type A/Type B behavior instruments.

Part Three

This part deals with the Inner World and scales that measure Self Esteem, Positive Outlook, Personal Power, Connection, Expression, and Compassion. Scales 13–16, Self Esteem, Positive Outlook, Personal Power, and Connection respectively, draw on cognitive therapy by Koabasa and Maddi's hardiness research, on Antonovsky's work on coherence, and on Wallston's locus-of-control studies. Scale 18, Compassion, stems from Spielberger and London's anger research.

Part Four

The final area involves Signals of Distress, which include physical, behavioral, and emotional problems. Physical Symptoms include many minor illnesses and symptoms such as back pain, headache, and upper respiratory infections. The Behavioral Symptoms are work avoidance, substance abuse, and eating disorders. The Emotional Symptoms include anxiety, depression, and obsessive-compulsive behavior. These scales are derived from the common stress-symptom checklist.

SUGGESTED READING

Borysenko, Joan. *Minding the Body, Mending the Mind*. New York: Addison-Wesley, 1987.

Brody, Jane. *Jane Brody's Nutrition Book: A Lifetime Guide to Eating for Better Health and Weight Control*. New York: Norton, 1981.

Burns, David D. *Feeling Good: The New Mood Therapy*. New York: Morrow, 1980.

Charlesworth, Edward A., and Ronald G. Nathan. *Stress Management*. New York: Ballantine, 1984.

Cooper, Robert K., Ph.D. *Health and Fitness Excellence: The Comprehensive Action Plan*. Boston: Houghton Mifflin, 1989.

———. *The Performance Edge*. Boston: Houghton Mifflin, 1991.

Cousins, Norman. *Anatomy of an Illness as Perceived by the Patient: Reflections on Healing and Regeneration*. New York: Norton, 1979.

Downing, George. *Massage and Meditation*. New York: Random House, 1974.

Dychtwald, Ken. *Bodymind*. New York: Bantam Books, 1977.

Friedman, Meyer, M.D., and Ray H. Rosenman, M.D. *Type A Behavior and Your Heart*. New York: Fawcett-Crest, 1974.

Gawain, Shakti. *Creative Visualization*. New York: Bantam, 1982.

Green, Elmer, and Alyce Green. *Beyond Biofeedback*. New York: Delacorte Press, 1977.

Johnson, Sonia. *Going Out of Our Minds: The Politics of Liberation*. Trumansburg, N.Y.: Crossing Press, 1987.

Justice, Blair. *Who Gets Sick: Thinking and Health*. Houston, Texas: Peak Press, 1987.

Lakein, Alexander. *How to Get Control of Your Time and Your Life*. New York: Signet, 1973.

Larson, B. *There's A Lot More to Health Than Not Being Sick*. Waco, Texas: Word Books, 1984.

Locke, Steven and Douglas Colligan. *The Healer Within: The New Medicine of Mind and Body*. New York: E.P. Dutton, 1986.

Mason, John L. *Stress Passages*. Berkeley, California: Celestial Arts, 1988.

Moody, R. A. Jr. *Laugh After Laugh: The Healing Power of Humor*. Jacksonville, Florida: Headwaters Press, 1978.

Sanford, Linda T. and Mary E. Donovan. *Women and Self-Esteem*. New York: Penguin, 1985.

Selye, Hans. *Stress of Life*. New York: McGraw Hill, 1976.

Witkin, Georgia, Ph.D. *The Female Stress Syndrome—Revised and Expanded Edition*. New York: Newmarket Press, 1991.

———. *The Male Stress Syndrome*. New York: Newmarket Press, 1985.

ABOUT ESTHER ORIOLI
AND ESSI SYSTEMS

Founded in 1983 in San Francisco by Esther Orioli, Essi Systems is an international stress research and consulting firm that specializes in helping companies and employees transform workplace stresses into opportunities for optimal performance. Essi's 1500 corporate clients, including AT&T, Bristol Meyers, Coca-Cola, and the State of Maine, use programs created by Essi Systems for organizational development, management leadership, and the enhancement of both company performance and job satisfaction. Essi Systems is currently studying the differences between how men and women experience stress in the workplace.

Esther Orioli, president of Essi Systems, is a well-known authority with more than 20 years experience in health research, management consulting, and medical-care cost containment. Before founding Essi Systems, Orioli was President and CEO of a San Francisco-based company that creates employee assistance programs, and before that served as Executive Director of a New York-based outpatient alcohol and drug treatment clinic. She holds a graduate degree in Adult Learning with a concentration in organizational systems, is a licensed alcoholism therapist, and a certified instructor for the U.S. Department of Health, Education, and Welfare.

Orioli and her colleagues spent six years testing and developing *StressMap,* and continue to collect data and conduct stress and performance research in Canada, Sweden, Japan, and the U.S.

Stress Management Books from Newmarket Press

Stressmap®: Personal Diary Edition—Expanded Edition
The Ultimate Stress Management, Self-Assessment and Coping Guide
Developed by Essi Systems
Foreword by Robert K. Cooper, Ph.D.

This stress measurement tool used by more than 1,500 companies, hospitals, and colleges integrates all major stress research—medical, psychological, and sociological—and gives you a revealing self-portrait of your stress health, from burn-out to optimal performance. The self-scoring questionnaire—which takes about an hour to complete—poses 300 questions about your environment, your inner world, your coping responses, and your own signals of stress overload. The "Action Planning Guide" gives more than 100 simply written, effective strategies for handling pressure on the job and at home.

The Female Stress Syndrome—Enlarged Second Edition
How to Become Stress-Wise in the 90s
Georgia Witkin, Ph.D.

Dr. Witkin was the first to document how and why women experience stress differently than men. Now, in this expanded edition, she addresses the increasing pressures in women's lives, from aging, AIDS, and infertility, to divorce, financial anxiety, and the corporate "glass ceiling." Included are checklists, quizzes, and a female stress questionnaire to help women identify sources of stress in their personal and public lives. Most importantly, Dr. Witkin identifies the symptoms of stress overload and provides practical short- and long-term coping strategies gleaned from more than fifteen years of clinical experience.

The Male Stress Syndrome—Updated Edition
How to Recognize and Live With It
Georgia Witkin, Ph.D.

Dr. Witkin explains why men develop the stress symptoms they do; how stress affects their bodies, careers, families, personal goals and expectations; and the differences between men and women coping with stress. She outlines the early warning signs of potentially harmful stress; provides checklists and profiles so that men can rate their own stress levels; and offers simple effective solutions including relaxation exercises for body and mind, in-depth stress management strategies, and sex therapy techniques.

Order from your local bookstore or send this coupon to
Newmarket Press, 18 East 48th Street, New York, NY 10017.

Please send me:

Qty.	Title	Format	Price	Total
_____	*StressMap®* (1-55704-081-8)	pb	$15.95	_____
_____	*Female Stress* (1-55704-098-2)	pb	$12.95	_____
_____	*Female Stress* (1-55704-099-0)	hc	$22.95	_____
_____	*Male Stress* (1-55704-205-5)	pb	$12.95	_____
		Subtotal		_____
		Shipping and handling*		_____
		Total amount enclosed		_____

I enclose a check or money order for $_____ payable to Newmarket Press.

NAME _____

ADDRESS _____

CITY/STATE/ZIP _____

*For postage and handling, add $2.50 for the first book, plus $1.00 for each additional book. Allow 4–6 weeks for delivery. Prices and availibility are subject to change.

Special discounts are available for orders of five or more copies. For information contact Newmarket Press, Special Sales Dept. 18 E. 48th St., NY, NY 10017;Tel.: 212–832–3575 or 800–669–3903; Fax: 212–832–3629

SM\BOBAD394.QXD